Paranoia

Paranoia

A Journey Into Extreme Mistrust and Anxiety

Daniel Freeman

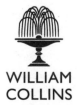

WILLIAM
COLLINS

William Collins
An imprint of HarperCollins*Publishers*
1 London Bridge Street
London SE1 9GF

WilliamCollinsBooks.com

HarperCollins*Publishers*
Macken House
39/40 Mayor Street Upper
Dublin 1
D01 C9W8, Ireland

First published in Great Britain in 2024 by William Collins

1

A catalogue record for this book is available from the British Library

ISBN 978-0-00-847258-0 (hardback)
ISBN 978-0-00-847259-7 (trade paperback)

Thank you for reading this book. It's important to note that it is not a medical textbook, and its contents are not a substitute for medical advice. Please always seek the advice of a qualified professional healthcare provider if you have questions or concerns about your own physical or mental health, and advise/support others to do so, too.

Typeset in Sabon MT by Palimpsest Book Production Ltd,
Falkirk, Stirlingshire

Printed and bound in the UK using
100% renewable electricity at CPI Group (UK) Ltd

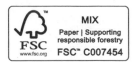

This book contains FSC™ certified paper and other controlled sources
to ensure responsible forest management.

For more information visit: www.harpercollins.co.uk/green

Contents

1.

Every day is a battle

In the summer of 2021, while I was working on the first drafts of this book, I published the results of a new treatment for persecutory delusions: the Feeling Safe programme. Persecutory delusions are the severest form of paranoia, which we can think of as *excessive mistrust of others in relation to the self*. They're very common in people diagnosed with schizophrenia. And they can wreck lives.

For me at least, publication of the data was a huge moment. Since first training as a clinical psychologist, my ambition has always been to provide new hope to patients by developing a treatment that is much better than the existing options. Feeling Safe, the product of three decades of researching and treating paranoia, marks the fulfilment of that ambition. Jane was one of the first patients to complete it. This is how things were for her before she began the Feeling Safe programme:

> I suffered with extremely debilitating paranoia and with voices that controlled my ability to be productive and that also regularly scared me. Though I am on strong medication the medication alone wasn't giving me enough help to feel safe. My life was a constant battle. I felt far too paranoid to participate in so many events and activities. I used to keep all my curtains shut and had all doors locked. I shut myself

away in my flat. I didn't feel my life was a life worth having really – I just felt there was a ticking time bomb till I got attacked or gave up myself.

A constant battle. A ticking time bomb. A life on hold. When I began my career as a clinical psychologist, I understood none of this. Let's rewind . . .

Secret signals

Autumn 1992. I am living with friends from university in the lee of HMP Brixton. The hulking Victorian prison has lately been much in the news, having failed to prevent two IRA inmates from escaping all the way to the Republic of Ireland. I have begun work at the Institute of Psychiatry (IoP), one of the largest centres in the world for mental health research. To mark the occasion, I've treated myself to a new jacket from Kensington Market, though already I'm beginning to worry that its shoulder pads are laughably large. Shoes duly shined, I'm a research assistant on one of the first clinical trials of psychological therapy for schizophrenia patients with delusions and hallucinations. (These experiences are also known as psychosis.) This is why I'm now struggling down a narrow, overgrown passageway in the front garden of a house in south London, squeezing past overflowing bins while brambles claw at my legs and arms and rain drives into my face. If anyone is watching – and I hope devoutly that they are not – they must take me for an incompetent burglar. This was definitely not mentioned in the job description. Surely, I think as I continue my slow progress to the back of the house, this can't be right. Why shouldn't I just present myself at the front door?

But the psychiatric nurse who briefed me was adamant that I shouldn't ring the doorbell. There would be no point: the man I have come to see would never appear. Robert believes that government agencies are conspiring to murder him. So instead of answering the door, Robert would be hiding in terror, keeping silent and still and crouching below window height. The only way to reach him is to give the secret signal: three knocks on the window at the side of the house. And so, feeling somewhat self-conscious, this is what I do. Sure enough, the kitchen door opens a fraction, Robert's apprehensive face appears, and I am politely hurried inside.

The house is dark and silent. Curtains are drawn; kitchen blinds closed. No radio plays. No music lightens the gloom. The place, like Robert, is on edge. It's as if the house is holding its breath, desperate not to give itself away. Straining to detect the disaster that one day – who knows, maybe today – is sure to come calling. Robert leads me down the murky hallway into a tiny living room. Actually, the room is not especially small – it just seems that way because it's so full of *stuff*. Every surface seems to be occupied. There are stacks of newspapers and books, towers of cassette cases, CDs and videos. Piles of neatly folded laundry lurk in unexpected corners. Even the carpet is covered with layers of rugs. In front of a large television is an armchair and beside the armchair is a small table on which sits a pile of *Radio Times*, mugs and cups, a half-full ashtray, and several packets of medication. Below on the carpet stand two jumbo-sized bottles of no-brand, generic cola. In the corner, a standard lamp supplies the only light in the house. Strikingly, what there isn't in this crammed and cluttered room is much in the way of decoration: no pictures on the bare walls, no photographs on the shelves, no souvenirs of happier times.

I introduce myself with what I hope is a friendly smile, but Robert meets my eye only briefly. 'Where shall I sit?' I ask brightly. With a mumbled apology, he clears some newspapers from an armchair and I lower myself into it. Robert lights a cigarette. His fingers, their tips yellowed by nicotine, tremble. In truth, we are probably both as nervous as each other. Robert is anxious because he is meeting a stranger. He doesn't see many people these days. He rarely leaves the house and relationships with family and friends have largely withered away over the years of isolation. Now he has to decide whether to open up to me. Can he trust this young guy he's only just met with his innermost thoughts and feelings? As for me, I'm still carrying around the baggage of my undergraduate experimental psychology reading. In schizophrenia, I was taught, we are beyond the pale of rationality – we're in the badlands of mental illness. Those who develop the disorder are therefore regarded as marginal too. As mental health professionals, we can't really relate to them as we would other patients. We shouldn't talk to them about their experiences. In my mind too are the warnings from my recent risk assessment training. Remain vigilant for possible trouble. Check for exits and position your chair accordingly.

But as Robert and I began to chat, I realised that the official version was nonsense. I saw that Robert could be eloquent and engaging, eminently capable of describing his feelings. And far from being irrational, those feelings made perfect sense in light of Robert's life experiences. It's a lesson that has guided my clinical work ever since. Whatever their situation, patients deserve clinicians' respect, attention and care. Patients' thoughts and emotions are important and meaningful and as therapists we are privileged to hear them. But we have to earn the right. We have to show that we can be trusted. That we are on their side. All this sounds obvious, I know. But as we'll see later in this book, people with psychosis haven't always been treated as they should by mental health professionals.

An infinite capacity for suspicion

Meeting Robert was my first encounter with persecutory delusions. But though my journey began with the severest type of paranoia, I've since learned that excessive mistrust is not confined to the psychiatric clinic. On the contrary, it is ubiquitous – it's the lens through which so many of us view the world. The proportion of people like Robert treated for schizophrenia or other psychotic conditions is small: around 1 per cent of the population. But that's the tip of the iceberg. They may never have been given a diagnosis, but somewhere between 1 and 3 per cent of people experience severe paranoia. Another 5 to 6 per cent of the population have delusions that are less severe but still distressing. And a further 10 to 15 per cent of people have regular, albeit milder, paranoid thoughts.

You don't need to be a clinical psychologist to notice how widespread extreme mistrust has become. Look at the prevalence of conspiracy beliefs. In 2020, as Covid-19's first wave wrought havoc across the world, I surveyed a representative sample of 2,501 adults in England. To my surprise and dismay, half of the participants endorsed at least one conspiracy theory. For instance, almost 50 per cent agreed to some extent with the idea that 'coronavirus is a bioweapon developed by China to destroy the West' and around one-fifth thought it possible that 'Jews have created the virus to collapse the economy for financial gain'. A quarter of respondents were receptive to the idea that the virus had been manufactured by the United Nations and World Health Organization (WHO) in order to take control. Around 17 per cent believed, at least to some degree, that vaccination safety data are often fabricated; that the authorities are covering up the harm that immunisation can cause children; and that the government is hiding a link between vaccination and autism. A further quarter of respondents were neutral in their opinion, which means that only around two-thirds of people outright rejected these conspiracy beliefs. Almost 24 per cent thought that human-induced climate change is a hoax. Given that 17 per cent neither agreed nor disagreed, it seems that only 60 per cent of people appear to accept the scientific consensus. Unlike paranoia, which is all about feeling personally threatened, conspiracy beliefs conjure a more general and diffuse harm. Typically, that imagined harm involves a powerful minority covertly mistreating the rest of us. But paranoia and conspiracy beliefs are both varieties of mistrust. Sure enough, the people in my survey who endorsed the conspiracy theories were also much more likely to display paranoid thinking.

The picture was no more encouraging in March 2023 when I surveyed more than ten thousand UK adults chosen to be representative for age, gender, ethnicity, income and region. Asked whether over the past month people had laughed at them behind their back, a third believed this somewhat or totally. Thirty-eight per cent said they were either somewhat or totally certain that people had done things to annoy them and 27 per cent that someone wanted to hurt them. Twenty-eight per cent had been distressed because of persecution.

Who's the rat?

'So *who's* the rat this time? I can say I definitely didn't do it, 'cause I know what I did or didn't do. But I can't definitely say that about anyone else 'cause I don't definitely know. For all I know, you're the rat.'

Reservoir Dogs (1992)

Meanwhile in 1992, while I'm meeting Robert the UK is still simmering after weeks of rioting across multiple towns and cities. It's a transatlantic echo of the disturbances in Los Angeles earlier that year following the acquittal of the Los Angeles Police Department officers who beat up Rodney King. In Sicily a car bomb kills the crusading anti-Mafia lawyer Paulo Borsellino, just a few weeks after his friend and colleague Giovanni Falcone met the same fate. In Wisconsin serial killer Jeffrey Dahmer is sentenced to life imprisonment for the murder of fifteen men. In July, three firebombs are discovered in the centre of Milton Keynes. At the end of October in London, IRA terrorists force a minicab to drive to Downing Street, where they detonate a bomb placed in the vehicle. (No one is hurt.) Meanwhile in the movies, a low-budget, blood-spattered gangster film by novice director Quentin Tarantino, *Reservoir Dogs*, opens in the US to modest box office interest.

In this context you may wonder what the problem is with mistrust. Isn't it a sensible response to a dangerous world? It's better to be vigilant than a victim, right? I'm not so certain. 'Survival,' wrote John le Carré, 'is an infinite capacity for suspicion.' But the character to whom he gives this line, Jim Prideaux, is an MI6 operative. Let's not live our lives like characters from a spy novel. (Infinite suspicion doesn't help Prideaux, who is betrayed by his best friend.) Let's choose a different narrative, a kinder way to make sense of our experiences. It's true, of course, that not everyone has our best interests at heart. Some threats, obviously, are real. And it would be naïve to accept as truth everything we read on the internet or indeed are told by those in power. But our wellbeing depends much less on suspicion than it does on the readiness to trust. I think Graham Greene was right: 'It is impossible to go through life without trust; that is to be imprisoned in the worst cell of all, oneself.'

So many of my patients have seen their lives poisoned by paranoia. Isolated from the rest of society, they are prey to depression, insomnia, anxiety. These are relatively extreme instances, for sure. But, as we will see in this book, the damage caused by mistrust doesn't stop at those with a diagnosis of psychosis. It's far more widespread than that. Like some invisible corrosive, it eats away at both individuals and society. So we need to reject mistrust. Clearly, there are times and places when it's wise to be wary. I wouldn't walk down a dark alleyway at night. I would likely estimate risk rather differently if I lived in, say, Kabul rather than in Oxford. But we must judge each situation on its own merits, guided by hard evidence rather than emotion. And unless there are very good grounds to think otherwise, we should start from the assumption that we are safe. Paranoia is essentially an interpretation of events. Although we may not appreciate it, there are always alternative explanations. In deciding what's going on, evidence is a much more reliable guide than fear. As the Russian proverb has it: *trust, but verify*. The alternative is to situate oneself in a world of jeopardy. It's to see life as a perpetual battle against an implacable foe. Like the doomed gangsters in *Reservoir Dogs*, it is to be tormented by the question: who is the rat?

Paranoia and anxiety

Despite the damage caused by excessive mistrust, and though society is increasingly ready to talk about mental health, paranoia tends to be overlooked as a clinical problem. As a result, it's mostly not well understood. (This is ironic given that the word 'paranoid' is constantly in use, typically as a synonym for 'afraid'.) Back in 1992, even among psychologists and psychiatrists there was scant interest in paranoia. As we'll see in Chapter 3, the problem was generally pigeonholed as a symptom of schizophrenia. Because schizophrenia is a disorder that affects a relatively small proportion of people, it was assumed that paranoia was similarly rare. Almost no one was concerned with understanding excessive mistrust in its own right: how it came about, what fuelled it, and what could be done to overcome it. Why should they be? What mattered, according to the then-conventional wisdom, was treating the patient's schizophrenia.

I reflected on my meeting with Robert while taking the bus back to the Institute of Psychiatry. The traditional account of paranoia started to strike me as unsatisfactory. It didn't fit with what I'd seen. And it didn't do justice to Robert's experiences. In fact, his behaviour reminded me of a much more everyday psychological problem than schizophrenia. By hiding away in the back of the house and only acknowledging callers who gave the special signal, Robert was trying to save himself from being killed or maimed. It was a textbook example of what I call a *defence*. In order to prevent ourselves or others from coming to some imagined harm, we modify our behaviour. We take precautions. The most common defence is simply to avoid the feared situation. But if that isn't possible we might make sure that someone else is with us, or avoid eye contact with other people, or dress inconspicuously.

Over the years I've learned that where there's paranoia, there are defensive behaviours. Pretty much every patient I see uses them. It's not a surprise. If you feel threatened, embattled, assailed by forces you can't hope to defeat, naturally you're going to do whatever you think will keep you safe. But it's not only people with persecutory delusions that use defences. The concept of 'safety-seeking behaviours' was developed by specialists in anxiety disorders – which, alongside depression, make up the majority of mental health cases. (Epidemiological studies have suggested that a third of people will experience an anxiety disorder at some point in their life: anxiety is everywhere.) Defences help people get through anxious situations. But they are a false friend. This is because what defences protect is not us, but our fears. They lock us into a narrative of threat because their use makes it impossible to judge whether we are truly in danger. The socially anxious woman who avoids speaking in meetings will never find out that, much to her surprise, no one laughs or yawns or demands to know who invited her in the first place. The man who crosses the street every time he spies a dog is deprived of the opportunity to discover whether his fear of being bitten is justified. And if Robert won't allow anyone in without the special kitchen-window knock, he will continue to assume that this is an essential precaution. Only by lowering our defences can we learn that our interpretation is flawed, that we are safer than we think. This isn't easy. Many of our defences will have taken root over several years. But unless we do so we will remain, at some level, in thrall to our fears.

Robert's defensive behaviour made me wonder whether paranoia might be better understood in terms of anxiety, rather than as some mysterious by-product of schizophrenia. Meeting him had provided another clue too. Robert had told me that his fears about the government played on his mind virtually non-stop, shaping his behaviour and affecting his mood. He worried about what might happen to him when he woke up in the morning; when he saw people walking or driving past the house; when he turned off the lights at night. 'I sometimes feel,' he'd said, 'as if I'm living in some kind of horror film. It's like there's no escape.' But this kind of all-consuming worry isn't as unusual as you might think. In fact it's a routine feature of anxiety disorders. Fearful of harm to ourselves or others – which is, fundamentally, what anxiety in all its diverse forms boils down to – our thoughts constantly gravitate towards the imagined catastrophe. We may suspect that we're getting things out of proportion. We may realise that there are more realistic ways of looking at the situation. And yet the pull of our worry is so powerful that it can seem impossible to resist.

Robert certainly looked anxious. Unfailingly polite, he was nevertheless often unable to focus fully on our conversation. Like a person with multiple diary commitments, Robert's attention was required elsewhere. Mostly, he seemed preoccupied with his own thoughts. He sat on the edge of his chair, tense as if ready to jump up at any moment. While we spoke, he appeared to be simultaneously processing the noises of the house, the sounds of the street outside. Most psychiatrists back then would have put Robert's anxious behaviour down to his persecutory delusions. He was fearful, they would have said, because he believed his life was in danger. To some extent, that interpretation was undoubtedly accurate. But what if there were more to it? Rather than being merely a side effect, could Robert's anxiety have played a part in *causing* his delusions? I wasn't thinking in terms of explaining the schizophrenia diagnosis. What fascinated me was Robert's paranoia. Even then it felt like a thread that might prove critical in the fabric of his mental health problems.

* * *

Meeting Robert had a profound effect on me. It prompted my first tentative steps towards truly understanding mistrust: why it develops; why it can be so difficult to shake off; how widespread it is; its impact on both individuals and society in general; how it fits into the psychological universe; and – most importantly – how it can be overcome.

To answer those questions, I've approached extreme mistrust with the same methodology I would use for any other psychological problem: producing a definition; charting the prevalence;

constructing and testing a theoretical model; and, based on that model, creating a carefully targeted therapy. I'll take you through this process in the coming chapters – rather like completing a jigsaw puzzle on fast forward. On that journey, we'll also explore the scale of mistrust in our society. We'll see how suspicion is rife, how conspiracy theories circulate like never before, and how all too often emotion trumps evidence. I'll show you how you can measure your own level of mistrust. And if it's higher than you'd like, what you can do to remedy things. Because although mistrust can seem ingrained, things can change for the better. The success of Feeling Safe proves that even those whose lives have been swallowed up by paranoia can learn to trust again. This is what has happened for Jane:

> My life is so incredibly different now . . . I am in control of my life now not my voices not my paranoia and not my worry but me. I know myself and can push myself far more than I ever have been able to previously. I am aiming to go to a festival soon something I have always wanted to do but never thought I'd be able to. My sleep is so good now. I have much better routines and as long as I stick to them my life flows better than it ever has.

Jane is now out and about, just as she wanted to be. Life is no longer the battle it once seemed. In the next chapter, we'll find out more about the treatment that helped her make this breakthrough.

2.

Feeling Safe

'I missed out on so many things in life. I missed out on meeting my friends, family events, meals, training, sports, I was just in a very paranoid state. Missed out on a lot of things. I lost contact with so many friends.'
Mason, Feeling Safe trial participant

In the thirty years since my encounter with Robert, I've met many other people whose paranoia is so overwhelming that they can scarcely leave the house. Unable to work, isolated from friends and family, almost half of patients with persecutory delusions are clinically depressed. This is a group that's really struggling. In fact, their psychological wellbeing often ranks in the lowest 2 per cent of the population. As if that weren't enough, people with persecutory delusions are more likely to develop a raft of serious but preventable physical problems, including high blood pressure, diabetes and heart disease. There are lots of reasons behind this, but one of them is undoubtedly the fact that it's incredibly difficult to maintain an active lifestyle and healthy diet when you're stuck at home and feeling low. You're just not in the right frame of mind to take care of yourself.

Robert had been taking antipsychotic medication, but it wasn't working well enough. I wish we'd been able to offer him the kind of psychological therapy that we can provide now. In my mind's eye, I imagine doing the sorts of exercises with him I've done so often with patients in recent years. I've managed, for example, to persuade him to stand with me on his doorstep – the one at the front of the house, the one he associates with disaster (with violent death, in fact).

'How are you feeling?' I ask after a couple of minutes.

Robert is scanning the street. His eyes dart left and right. He's shifting from foot to foot, as if the ground beneath him is red hot.

'Um. I'm nervous, to be honest. My body feels wired. Buzzy. There are quite a few people walking down the street.'

'What's running through your mind about them?'

He smiles grimly. 'Well, that man and woman over there showed up as soon as I opened the door. It's like they were waiting for me. So I'm wondering what they're up to.'

'What do you think they might do?'

'I dunno. But I feel like I should keep an eye on them.'

'How about signs of safety? Do you see any of those?'

Robert looks around. 'Um. Over by the bus stop – that woman with the toddler.'

'You think she might be okay?'

'Yeah, she's got her child with her. She's not looking towards me. She's just going about her business.'

'Good. And the lady over there – the one who's just walked past the house?'

'Yeah. I saw her. I thought she was okay. But then I think she did look round. So I'm not sure if she was looking at someone else.'

'Okay. Is there anything bad happening?'

There is a pause. Robert seems to be carefully considering his reply. 'Well, no one is doing anything bad right now.'

'How does your body feel?'

'It's hard to describe. Like sort of racing inside. But it's not as bad as when we first came out.'

'So your body is telling you there's danger. But otherwise what *is* going on?'

'Um. Well, there's not much, is there? People walking past occasionally. A little queue for the bus at the end of the road. Not much. Mind you, that guy has just stopped near the house so I dunno what he's doing.'

'And now?'

Robert smiles. 'Yeah. As soon as I said that, he's carried on walking. So yeah, I guess it's sort of alright.'

'Let's just stand here for a little bit and see what happens.'

Robert nods. He's still looking up and down the street, but his face doesn't seem quite so taut with tension. He's moved a little further forward too.

'Let's refocus on the safety now,' I say after a minute or so. 'What signs are there? What nice things are there?'

'I dunno. It's an alright street, I suppose. I quite like it. It's got loads of trees. Just normal really – which is good, I think. People just doing their thing. No one's really paying us much attention. It's actually almost quite calm. Everyday life. Yeah.'

'How's your body in terms of the danger signals?'

'Um. Much calmer than it was. Still sort of switched on a little. A bit ready, just in case. But it's come down.'

'And the thoughts about harm happening?'

'Well, I can't see anyone at the moment who looks like they might cause a problem. It seems alright at the minute. Yeah. It seems okay.'

The long road

'[Feeling Safe] gives you a companion to share something. That's where it begins because most of the people with these kind of psychotic things, the first thing they do is they don't know who to share with.'

Rajiv, Feeling Safe patient

Back in 1992, hardly anyone had received cognitive behavioural therapy (CBT) for persecutory delusions. Robert was one of the first – he, like the research, was a trailblazer. That I happened to be working on the trial was a stroke of luck. In those days, schizophrenia was generally understood as a biological disorder: the result of a physical problem with the brain. Psychological perspectives didn't really get a look in. That was certainly how the topic was addressed during my undergraduate degree, though even then it had seemed to me a strangely reductive approach. To my great fortune, the trial brought me into the orbit of a group of pioneering clinical researchers: Philippa Garety, Elizabeth Kuipers, David Fowler, Paul Bebbington and Graham Dunn. I sometimes wonder what I'd be doing now if my application to be their research assistant had been unsuccessful.

CBT for psychosis can certainly reduce paranoia, but for many people the benefits are modest. Nevertheless, in terms of mental health care it's been a game-changer. In the early trials, we usually worked with long-term patients, people the psychiatrists had given up on. The fact that psychological therapy could help in these cases was a big breakthrough, not only for the patients but for mental health professionals too. The idea that psychotherapy might benefit people with psychosis began to seem less far-fetched. (And if it could help these patients, what might it do for people whose problems weren't so ingrained?)

Yet for all the promise of CBT for psychosis, I was sure we could do better. How? What might move us forward? For me, it was the relationship between mistrust and anxiety that really opened the door. Paranoia can't be reduced to anxiety, but recognising the similarities brings into play an incredibly rich storehouse of clinical knowledge and effective techniques. Because although anxiety problems are extremely common, they are also treatable. The best psychological therapies start from the insight that anxiety is a response to perceived danger. Sometimes, of course, that perception is correct and the threat is real. That's why anxiety is adaptive: it can keep us alive. But not always. On occasion we get things wrong. We overestimate the likely threat. When that happens, anxiety ceases to be useful. In fact, it can be hugely disruptive – both in terms of our emotions (fear, worry, sadness) and our behaviour (think of Robert hiding away from the world). And all of it entirely unnecessary.

The remedy for anxiety problems is to help the patient learn that, despite what they may assume, they are safe. And it turns out that this approach is an extremely powerful way of overcoming paranoia too. The best way for the patient to learn they are safe is by experience. It means getting out there rather than staying in. Not discussing an activity in a consulting room, but actually trying it. And doing so without using defensive strategies. In time the person's anxieties are crowded out by new memories of safety. Now this can be a gruelling process for patients. We don't throw them straight in at the deep end. I wouldn't start by asking someone like Robert, who's been more or less housebound for years, to test out his fears by taking a rush-hour trip on the London Underground. Instead, I work with my patients to design a programme of activities that gradually increases in difficulty.

All the same, I'm asking people to attempt things they'd ordinarily avoid. Many patients have been experiencing persecutory thoughts every day for years – decades in some cases. Their fears are so deeply rooted that the patient can scarcely recall a time before the fears were present, nor believe that one day they could be gone.

Crucially, patients are often dealing too with a range of problems and experiences that block the new learning we're aiming for. Perhaps they have been treated badly by other people and feel vulnerable as a consequence. If you've been bullied as a child, for instance, being wary of other people is an understandable response. Memories of that mistreatment may be continuing to upset them. They may be spending a lot of time worrying. They're probably avoiding the places that trigger their paranoid thoughts. Sleep problems are common, as is low self-esteem. These 'maintenance factors' spark and strengthen persecutory delusions. So we're not going to get far treating paranoia unless we deal with these other problems. Rather than being overwhelmed by their fears, we need to help people get into a psychological state that allows new learning to happen.

Feeling Safe is built on these two fundamental insights: that safety must be learned through practical experience and that this is most likely to happen when we sort out the other problems stoking a patient's paranoia. Arriving at these insights and constructing a fully fledged therapy required years of effort. First, we needed to refine and rigorously test our new understanding of the causes of persecutory delusions. Next, we built and evaluated brief interventions to tackle each of those causes and show whether this affected people's paranoia. I then had to figure out how to combine those interventions into the new six-month treatment. Finally, we needed to test that treatment. Patients were a crucial part of the design process. And we would not have got far without a succession of UK mental health funders – the National Institute for Health Research (NIHR), the Medical Research Council (MRC) and the Wellcome Trust – stepping up to the plate. But what's it actually like to undertake the Feeling Safe programme? If you came to my clinic for treatment or (as is often the case) I and a colleague visited you at home, what could you expect?

Assessment time

As with any health intervention, my first step is to check whether the treatment is right for the individual. What problems do they want help with? Are they difficulties Feeling Safe is best placed to tackle? If so, does the person want to give it a go? Invariably people are pointed in my direction by their psychiatric team. But I still want to take the time to explain the therapy – to be as transparent as possible. And I want to discover exactly what difficulties the person is experiencing.

I begin by asking them to describe a recent experience of paranoia. (Some people live with almost constant paranoia, in which case I'll suggest they focus on a particular recent moment.) One woman told me she'd lain awake the previous night worrying that poison gas was being pumped into her flat. Often the situation is more prosaic: feeling afraid while out shopping, for example. Sometimes it's the journey to the therapy session that sparks the fear. I want as many details as possible. So we play it out, moment by moment: 'Let's start at the beginning. What were you doing just before you stepped out of your front door to come here?' I draw out the context, the psychological processes, the decision-making. And, to be sure we're both on the same page, I summarise what I'm hearing and how it seems to me. 'So, you saw the man at the bus stop staring at you nastily? It meant that something bad was about to happen? That must have been really unsettling for you. But of course people often look in the direction of others. What made the look nasty?'

I am striving to see the world through the patient's eyes – to walk for a while in their shoes. This is the key part of the assessment and it's the element I like best. If I get it right, the person feels understood. They're more confident that they're working with a skilled professional. And together we've put in place a framework to guide the treatment over the weeks and months to come. There's an additional benefit too. Therapists working with people who have persecutory delusions sometimes worry that they'll become objects of fear themselves. But when we're curious and caring about a patient's experiences, and candid about how we see their situation and what can be done to improve it, it's not paranoia that is fostered: it's trust.

Typically, I'll devote the first sixty-minute meeting to explaining the therapy, conducting the initial assessment and setting some high-level goals. Unless the patient wants more time on these preliminaries, my priority is to get on with active learning. To set a direction and begin the process of positive change. This is a much quicker therapeutic pace than usual for people with psychosis. But I know I'll have ample opportunity to ask questions and refine my view as the sessions progress. And as we get to know one another better, that conversation tends to become increasingly open. One other reason I can get to the active therapy fast is that I'll already have seen the questionnaires the person has completed before the first session. Questionnaires play a key part in assessing most mental health problems. The best of them have been developed by testing with hundreds of patients and thousands of other people from the general population. But when I began researching paranoia, I couldn't find a high-quality assessment tool. Those that did exist were now pretty dated. They weren't based on a clear definition of the problem. So we badly needed a new questionnaire, one that reflected our new understanding of paranoia. This meant, among other things, sensitivity to the broad spectrum of paranoia rather than just the most severe instances. That ground-breaking assessment tool was developed in 2007. The work was led by Catherine Green, a student of Philippa Garety's, Elizabeth Kuipers' and mine at the Institute of Psychiatry. After a decade of use, and having obtained data from thousands of people, we were able to revise the questionnaire to improve it, and you can try it now (see Table 1). As you answer the questions, think back to your experiences over the past month.

Table 1 Part A	Not at all		Somewhat		Totally
1 I spent time thinking about friends gossiping about me.	0	1	2	3	4
2 I often heard people referring to me.	0	1	2	3	4
3 I have been upset by friends and colleagues judging me critically.	0	1	2	3	4
4 People definitely laughed at me behind my back.	0	1	2	3	4
5 I have been thinking a lot about people avoiding me.	0	1	2	3	4
6 People have been dropping hints for me.	0	1	2	3	4
7 I believed that certain people were not what they seemed.	0	1	2	3	4
8 People talking about me behind my back upset me.	0	1	2	3	4

Table 1 Part B	Not at all		Somewhat		Totally
1 Certain individuals have had it in for me.	0	1	2	3	4
2 People wanted me to feel threatened, so they stared at me.	0	1	2	3	4
3 I was sure certain people did things in order to annoy me.	0	1	2	3	4
4 I was convinced there was a conspiracy against me.	0	1	2	3	4
5 I was sure someone wanted to hurt me.	0	1	2	3	4
6 I couldn't stop thinking about people wanting to confuse me.	0	1	2	3	4
7 I was distressed by being persecuted.	0	1	2	3	4
8 It was difficult to stop thinking about people wanting to make me feel bad.	0	1	2	3	4
9 People have been hostile towards me on purpose.	0	1	2	3	4
10 I was angry that someone wanted to hurt me.	0	1	2	3	4

To calculate your score, simply add up the totals for each part of the questionnaire. Scores of 0–9 for Part A and 0–5 for Part B are in the normal range. People with an elevated level of paranoia typically score 10–15 on Part A and 6–10 on Part B. Scoring 21–24 on Part A and 18–27 on Part B indicates severe paranoia – the kind that most of my Feeling Safe patients present with.

Using a market research company, I gave this questionnaire to a representative sample of the UK adult population in March 2023. Table 2 shows how those ten thousand people scored:

Table 2 Part A	Not at all		Somewhat		Totally
1 I spent time thinking about friends gossiping about me.	50%	16%	16%	12%	6%
2 I often heard people referring to me.	51%	18%	15%	11%	5%
3 I have been upset by friends and colleagues judging me critically.	48%	17%	16%	13%	7%
4 People definitely laughed at me behind my back.	50%	16%	13%	12%	8%
5 I have been thinking a lot about people avoiding me.	49%	16%	15%	13%	9%
6 People have been dropping hints for me.	57%	15%	13%	10%	5%
7 I believed that certain people were not what they seemed.	34%	16%	19%	17%	14%
8 People talking about me behind my back upset me.	44%	15%	15%	14%	13%

Table 2 Part B	Not at all		Somewhat		Totally
1 Certain individuals have had it in for me.	49%	16%	16%	11%	8%
2 People wanted me to feel threatened, so they stared at me.	60%	12%	12%	10%	5%
3 I was sure certain people did things in order to annoy me.	46%	17%	16%	13%	9%
4 I was convinced there was a conspiracy against me.	61%	12%	12%	10%	6%
5 I was sure someone wanted to hurt me.	62%	12%	11%	9%	7%
6 I couldn't stop thinking about people wanting to confuse me.	60%	13%	12%	10%	6%

7 I was distressed by being persecuted.	61%	12%	12%	10%	6%
8 It was difficult to stop thinking about people wanting to make me feel bad.	56%	13%	13%	10%	7%
9 People have been hostile towards me on purpose.	54%	14%	13%	11%	8%
10 I was angry that someone wanted to hurt me.	59%	12%	12%	10%	8%

Like I say, there's an awful lot of mistrust around.

Of course, we're not just keen to measure paranoia. We also want to find out if the person is experiencing other difficulties that make it hard to learn that they're safe. We have a much better chance of dealing with someone's persecutory delusions if we can first make progress with these additional problems. In Feeling Safe, patients get to choose from modules designed to improve sleep, reduce worry, boost self-confidence, help them cope better with hearing voices, and make new learning about safety. Why these modules? Well, from clinical experience I knew these were common issues for people with persecutory delusions – issues for which they wanted (but seldom received) treatment. They were plausible factors in the development and maintenance of paranoia. And they were problems I was confident we could tackle with psychological therapy.

To follow up on these insights from my clinical work, together with the main Feeling Safe trial we conducted a large survey with 1,800 people being treated in services for psychosis. Of the patients with persecutory delusions, almost 80 per cent were worrying excessively. Sixty-five per cent were sleeping badly; a similar proportion frequently heard voices. Almost 54 per cent reported very low psychological wellbeing and a similar proportion had a strongly negative view of themselves. We asked the patients what they would most like help with. Again, of those with severe paranoia three-quarters wanted to worry less; over 70 per cent wanted to feel happier, safer and more self-confident; two-thirds were keen to improve their decision-making; 64 per cent wanted to be more active; and a similar number wanted to sleep better, and to cope better with their voices.

Alongside the assessment conversation, we use a range of questionnaires to help decide which modules a patient might want to tackle. You can try some of them now. First up is the Oxford Positive Self Scale (Table 3), a questionnaire we devised to gauge how people feel about themselves. If you'd like to complete this short version, focus on the past seven days. To work out your score, just add up your marks – which could be a maximum of 32. The higher it is, the more self-confident you are. A score of 16 or under puts people among the lowest third of the population for levels of positive self-belief.

Table 3	Do not believe it	Believe it slightly	Believe it moderately	Believe it very much	Believe it totally
1 I can succeed.	0	1	2	3	4
2 I am worthwhile.	0	1	2	3	4
3 I rise to the challenge.	0	1	2	3	4
4 I can do things as well as anyone else.	0	1	2	3	4
5 I can relax.	0	1	2	3	4
6 I can have fun.	0	1	2	3	4
7 I am a good person.	0	1	2	3	4
8 I am helpful.	0	1	2	3	4

Another measure we developed is the Dunn Worry Questionnaire (see Table 4). It's named after the late Graham Dunn, a wonderful methodologist and statistician – and a mentor for me – who died in 2019. Graham helped work on the psychometric techniques used to compile the questionnaire. Base your answers on your experiences over the past month. A total score of 21 or more suggests clinically high levels of worry.

Table 4	None of the time	Rarely	Some of the time	Often	All of the time
1 I've been worrying a lot.	0	1	2	3	4
2 In my mind I have been going over problems again and again.	0	1	2	3	4
3 There was little I could do to stop worrying.	0	1	2	3	4
4 I have been worrying even though I didn't want to.	0	1	2	3	4
5 Worry has stopped me focusing on important things in my day.	0	1	2	3	4
6 Worry has stopped me sleeping.	0	1	2	3	4
7 Worry has caused me to feel upset.	0	1	2	3	4
8 Worry has made me feel stressed.	0	1	2	3	4
9 Worry has made me feel anxious.	0	1	2	3	4
10 Worry has made me feel hopeless.	0	1	2	3	4

Our offer to patients is straightforward: we are experts at helping people feel safer. That in turn will make you happier and allow you to do more of what's important to you. The patient decides what those activities are. They set the goal: what is it they'd like to be able to accomplish that they can't do now? For some people the objective is as basic as leaving the house. For others it might be taking public transport, seeing friends and family, or getting back to education or work. How many – and which – modules they tackle is their choice. That said, I encourage everyone to complete the Feeling Safer module. It's the cornerstone of the therapy: the module that focuses on learning safety. Typically, patients work through two or three additional modules over the six months of the programme. Every week they meet with a therapist, who they can also contact by text and phone. We organise regular calls in between sessions. Meanwhile, patients undertake homework practising the techniques they've learned in the face-to-face meetings. It can be pretty full-on. But we aim to be alongside the patient throughout the process. And the results can be life-changing.

Mason's story

'[I was] too paranoid about going out. Thinking that someone's going to stab me or start a fight. So I was housebound. I missed out on a lot of family events. I'd be very shy. I'd stay in my room when visitors would come to the home. Purely paranoia. . . . I couldn't sleep. And when you've been without sleep for two or three days you start hallucinating. It's quite horrible. Sleeping in the day from 9 a.m. to 5 p.m., which is the time people are working and I'm asleep. I'd wake up and during the winter it was dark – so I'd slept through the daylight. There was so much worry on my mind that I couldn't sleep. I'd lie in bed, and I'd

*be thinking: "Tomorrow something's going to happen". It would
play on my mind 24/7. I couldn't enjoy the things I used to.'*

Mason, though a very talented person, had been at an
extremely low ebb before beginning the Feeling Safe treatment.
Having struggled with paranoia for several years, by the time
we met Mason had withdrawn from the world. Holding down
a job had become impossible. So too was any form of social
life. It was all simply too frightening. He spent his days in his
bedroom, sleeping at all hours and worrying when awake.

Initially Mason had been dubious about Feeling Safe.
Committing to a long and demanding course of treatment
requires energy and resilience. Understandably, he wasn't sure
he had much of either. When he did eventually sign up, there
was no miraculous overnight transformation. Progress was
gradual, as it often is. As therapists, we must find the pace that
fits the patient. But Mason was determined and, step by step,
he moved forward: 'Initially I was housebound, and the therapist would come visit my home. We'd have a chat and build up
trust and rapport. It took a while but eventually I got convinced
to go for short walks. The short walks were great. They helped
me lift my paranoia.' Building rapport with patients is critical.
But it can take time. Many psychosis patients have been in the
mental healthcare system for decades and feel they have little
that is positive to show for it. They can be cautious, sceptical,
reserved. Like many Feeling Safe patients, Mason emphasised
the importance of forming a strong relationship with his therapist: 'Talking to someone who can understand you after building
trust is just brilliant. Really brilliant.'

As with all the Feeling Safe patients, I conducted an initial
assessment with Mason. Present too was a clinical psychologist
from my team. Mason was immediately likeable: warm, friendly
and witty. The assessment helped us identify the first treatment

target, which Mason and the clinical psychologist worked on in the next sessions. After six weeks we all met to review how things had gone and discuss which module to tackle next. Given the chaotic state of Mason's sleep, getting that sorted out was a priority for him. Disrupted sleep is extremely common among patients with severe paranoia. And, as you might imagine, it really doesn't help. Mason had fallen into the habit of staying up later and later. With little to do, his worries had free rein. Sitting in his chair, lying fretting on his bed, by the time evening came around Mason didn't feel tired. It was only early in the morning that he would finally drift off. Basically, he'd turned the normal sleep–wake cycle on its head. He was awake when almost everyone else was asleep – which only fuelled a sense of isolation. When we first got started with therapy, the sessions had to be scheduled for late in the day: in the morning he wasn't sufficiently awake and alert.

So we worked with Mason to gradually adjust his sleep routine. The first step was to agree upon a set time to wake up. Gradually, we moved that time earlier in the day. And we made sure that an increasing proportion of those extra daytime hours were spent being active. Getting up earlier, and doing more during the day, made it easier for Mason to fall asleep at night. Learning to feel better about himself, and to handle stress and worry, helped too:

The sleep therapy was superb. [I had been] Going to bed at 5 a.m. and waking at 1 p.m. And slowly cut it back by doing more things and activities in the day. Building confidence – another big thing the therapist helped with. Building confidence and being active in the day. Because the reward is a better sleep. It makes a massive difference to feeling paranoid if you have good sleep.

Encouraged by the progress he'd made with the sleep work,

Mason threw himself into the other parts of the programme, including of course the central Feeling Safe module. Six months later the change was remarkable:

> I had a bit of an epiphany. I thought: I'm around so many people and I don't feel angry or paranoid. I genuinely do feel safe. I don't think someone is going to harm me in any way – not in the long term or in the short term. It worked. It really did. It helped massively. You get better sleep, feel more confident, be more active in the day.
>
> Genuinely, inside I feel very happy. It's profoundly changed my life. I don't have to worry any more about people potentially attacking me or thinking sometimes there's a weapon in their pocket. That's all kind of floated away.

The trial

Mason was one of 130 participants in Feeling Safe's clinical trial, which ran from early 2016 to the summer of 2020. The anecdotal evidence from patients and therapists alike had been encouraging, but would the numbers bear that out? I had no idea until the statisticians' analysis, around two months after the last patient had finished their final follow-up assessments. It was a nerve-wracking period, ratcheting up as the day of the big reveal – the statisticians analysis – approached. Every morning, and with mounting anxiety, I wondered: will this be the day that the email arrives?

I had wanted to produce a psychological therapy for paranoia that would work for 50 per cent of patients for whom anti-psychotic medication had failed. That was a goal we exceeded. Half of patients at the end of treatment no longer had a persecutory delusion. A further quarter experienced moderate benefit.

And those gains were still largely present when we checked in with our patients six months after they had completed treatment. Feeling Safe didn't only tackle paranoia. It also brought a big improvement in patients' general wellbeing. And it was very popular: almost everyone stayed the course, which is unusual for an intensive six-month programme. I like to think that people attended so assiduously because of the usefulness of the intervention, and the kindness and attentiveness of our therapists.

These kinds of results made Feeling Safe by some distance the most effective psychological treatment for persecutory delusions. As I looked at the 130 people, their testimonies and their requests to continue with therapy, it felt clear that the treatment could help many, many more. The challenge became to make it available to the many thousands of people whose lives have been variously disrupted by paranoia.

But if psychological therapy can make such a difference to people with persecutory delusions, why has it taken so long to get here? Why were persecutory delusions of such little interest to previous generations of clinicians and researchers? What did they think was going on with their patients?

3.

A short history of paranoia

'I seek, sir, God bless you, for a gentleman that talks besides
to himself when he's alone, as if he were in Bedlam . . .'
John Webster and Thomas Dekker, *Northward Ho* (1607)

Bethlem Royal Hospital in London is the world's oldest psychiatric facility, with six 'insane' men recorded as living there in 1403. It emerged from the priory of St Mary of Bethlehem, which was founded in 1247 on the site of today's Liverpool Street Station. In due course 'Bethlehem' became known as 'Bethlem' – and also 'Bedlam', the latter term soon (and still) being used to denote any scene of madness and confusion. In 1948 the advent of the National Health Service brought Bethlem, now situated in suburban southeast London, into partnership with another famous psychiatric hospital, the Maudsley. Allied to the two was a new mental health research centre, the Institute of Psychiatry. The IoP is where I cut my teeth as a clinical psychologist and where I developed many of the theoretical ideas about paranoia that were eventually to underpin Feeling Safe. I worked at the IoP for almost twenty years, undertaking research and treating patients both at the Maudsley and at Bethlem Royal. A battered old minibus ferried staff back and forth on a 45-minute journey between the two hospitals.

Much of my research and clinical practice was focused then,

as it is now, on patients with a diagnosis of schizophrenia – and especially the persecutory delusions that are so common in this group. Aware of how little I knew about the subject, very early into my time at the IoP I resolved to rectify that deficit. I learned so much from patients, supervisors, mentors, peers, and read everything I could lay my hands on. Each morning on the way to my office I would leaf through the immaculate new journals laid out on a table upstairs in the Institute's library. Each evening I would descend the spiral staircase into the library basement where the old books and journals were housed. The ceiling was low, the light was patchy and artificial. My hands were soon covered with dust. Winding a handle opened the shelving units, and drastically shrank the aisle space. I wondered whether anyone had ever become jammed between yellowing stacks of *The Lancet* or the *Journal of Nervous and Mental Disease*. It seemed unlikely. Traffic down there was sparse. But as I educated myself about the paranoia with which my patients were now battling, I was fascinated (and often aghast) to discover how such experiences had been regarded in the past. It turned out that there was a local connection too. Bethlem had been home to James Tilly Matthews, the subject of one of the first published accounts of the condition eventually called schizophrenia: John Haslam's *Illustrations of Madness*, which appeared in 1810. Haslam worked as the hospital's apothecary – what we would call today a pharmacist, though his role in patient care extended far beyond simply dispensing medication. (Like Bethlem's other medical officers, however, Haslam doesn't seem to have spent huge amounts of time in the hospital. He told a House of Commons committee in 1815 that he usually arrived at 11 a.m., then 'stays half an hour, or sometimes longer than that'.) Central to *Illustrations of Madness* were Matthews' sustained and terrifying persecutory delusions.

The Air Loom

Matthews was first confined to Bethlem in January 1797. In those days the hospital was located in Moorfields, just north of the City of London. Around two hundred psychiatric patients were accommodated in often brutal conditions. Bethlem's rules stated that 'none of the Officers or Servants shall at any time beate or abuse any of the Lunatickes'. These stipulations, however, were routinely flouted. Those tasked with caring for the patients could be cruel, callous and corrupt. Mental, physical and sexual abuse was not uncommon. Restraint was seen as a legitimate means of control. In one notorious case during Haslam's time at the hospital, James Norris was kept chained up for twelve years: 'A stout iron ring was riveted around his neck, from which a short chain passed through a ring made to slide upwards and downwards on an upright massive iron bar, more than six feet high, inserted into the wall.' Bethlem's governors insisted that Norris's treatment had been 'on the whole merciful and humane'.

Haslam tells us little about Matthews' life before arriving at Bethlem. There is, for example, no record of his age in 1797, but we do know that he was born in Wales; that he was married with two children; and that he had worked as a tea merchant. Matthews' paranoia had led directly to his incarceration in Bethlem. Haslam recounts, for example, 'that in some apartment near London Wall, there is a gang of villains profoundly skilled in Pneumatic Chemistry, who assail him by means of an Air Loom'. Among the dozens of horrors reportedly inflicted by this imaginary device on Matthews (and other supposed victims) were:

Kiteing . . . As boys raise a kite in the air, so these wretches, by means of the air-loom and magnetic impregnations, contrive to lift into the brain some particular idea, which floats and undulates in the intellect for hours together; and how much soever the person assailed may wish to direct his mind to other objects, and banish the idea forced upon him, he finds himself unable . . .

Lobster-cracking. This is an external pressure of the magnetic atmosphere surrounding the person assailed, so as to stagnate his circulation, impede his vital motions, and produce instant death.

Bomb-bursting . . . The fluid which resides in the brain and nerves, the vapor floating in the blood-vessels, and the gaz which occupies the stomach and intestines, become highly rarified and rendered inflammable, occasioning a very painful distension over the whole body. Whilst the assailed person is thus labouring, a powerful charge of the electrical battery (which they employ for this purpose) is let off, which produces a terrible explosion, and lacerates the whole system.

Matthews believed that he was not the only person in danger. Even before his admission to Bethlem, he had warned anyone who would listen that numerous gangs, each equipped with an Air Loom, were operating across London. Not only this, but gang members were busy 'impregnating' citizens with the 'magnetic fluid' that rendered them vulnerable to the effects of the Loom: 'In consequence of the numerous gangs established in this metropolis, all the persons holding high situations in the government are held impregnated. . . . their opinions would be communicated to the enemy on the subjects of peace, commercial intercourse, or the fitting out of armaments.'

Convinced that these gangs were aiding France in the Napoleonic wars of the 1790s, Matthews had alerted the British government. A constant flow of warning letters to ministers was supplemented by regular visits to their offices. Perhaps predictably, these efforts merely resulted in his hospitalisation. Matthews was adamant that he was the victim of a conspiracy. He protested that the gangs had persuaded the authorities that he was insane 'for the purpose of plunging me into a madhouse, to invalidate all I said, and for the purpose of confining me within the measure of the Bedlam-attaining-airloom-warp. . . . so as to overpower my reason and speech, and destroy me in their own way, while all should suppose it was insanity which produced my death.' (The idea that psychiatric admission is part of a plot is something I often hear from patients.) Once confined in Bethlem, Matthews alleged that he was subject to regular telepathic communication from the gangs.

Matthews did not leave Bethlem until 1814. Even then, his destination was another asylum, where he died a year later. His relatives, who had never accepted that he was mentally ill, had brought his case to the courts in 1809, presenting to them assessments from two doctors. Their efforts were unsuccessful. Haslam reported: 'There are already too many maniacs allowed to enjoy a dangerous liberty, and the Governors of Bethlem Hospital, confiding in the skill and integrity of their medical officers, were not disposed to liberate a mischievous lunatic to disturb the good order and peace of society.'

Para-nous

Haslam's vivid portrayal of James Tilly Matthews' paranoia was novel, but of course the experience he described was not. As for the word 'paranoia', that dates back all the way to ancient Greece, though it then meant something rather different. The physician Hippocrates, born on the island of Kos around 460

BCE, coined the term to denote the delirium sometimes caused by a very high temperature. He put together the Greek words for 'beside' (*para*) and 'mind' (*nous*) to create a word that literally meant 'out of one's mind'. Such delirium might include fears about other people, but Hippocrates' 'paranoia' encompassed the fever in all its manifestations. In any case, the word soon drifted out of the ancient medical lexicon and into common usage as a synonym for 'crazy' or 'insane'. You can find it used in this way in works by Euripides, Aeschylus, Aristophanes, Aristotle and Plato. Other ancient Greek writers used the term to denote senility. But absent from all of these prototypical paranoias is any connotation of threat from other people.

For centuries the term fell into disuse. But it made a comeback in 1763 when the French physician and scholar François Boissier de Sauvages de Lacroix (1706–67) published *Nosologia Methodica*, the first attempt at a scientific classification of diseases. (Sauvages worked on the *Nosologia* for more than thirty years in 'an endless cycle of revision and editions'. Its final incarnation ran to ten volumes, each of more than five hundred pages.) This was a period of growing interest in mental illness and Sauvages devoted a significant proportion of his book to the topic. Rather like Hippocrates, Sauvages used the term 'paranoia' to describe the kind of derangement brought upon by a high fever, but he also broadened it to cover dementia. Nevertheless, 'paranoia' still denoted a problem with clear physical causes.

The nineteenth century saw the rise of the new discipline of psychiatry, with the very first chair in the discipline established at Leipzig University in 1811. And it was the first incumbent of that chair, Johann Heinroth (1777–1843), who began to use the word 'paranoia' interchangeably with the term *Verrücktheit* (madness) to describe a wide range of delusional thoughts (including, for example, ideas about the supernatural and a kind of megalomania). As with earlier incarnations, 'paranoia' still lacked the specificity of personal threat. But it wasn't entirely business as usual, because for Heinroth delusions were essentially *psychological* phenomena. (Heinroth believed that mental illness was primarily an affliction of the soul. The therapeutic task of psychiatrists was to help patients adopt a Christian way of life.)

Gradually, the use of 'paranoia' to describe delusions became widely accepted. Writing in 1911, the influential Swiss psychiatrist Eugen Bleuler (1857–1939) – the person who pioneered the terms 'schizophrenia' and 'autism', among others – defined paranoia as:

> The construction, from false premises, of a logically developed and in its various parts logically connected, unshakeable delusional system without any demonstrable disturbance affecting any of the other mental functions and, therefore, also without any symptoms of 'deterioration,' if one ignores the paranoiac's complete lack of insight into his own delusional system.

Like Heinroth's before him, Bleuler's 'paranoia' meant irrational, illogical, unfounded thoughts. And again, though those thoughts might concern persecution, the term was not exclusive: all types of delusion were included. English-speaking psychiatrists could be cutting about the catch-all use of 'paranoia' by their German colleagues. Writing in 1892, Hack Tuke lamented: 'It is regarded as synonymous with that very favourite word of the German alienists "Verrucktheit", in respect of which there has been so much difference of opinion and so much change . . . that a lamentable amount of confusion and obscurity has been introduced into the nomenclature of mental alienation.' Amid the confusion, however, a consensus was emerging – and it was not good news for people experiencing persecutory delusions.

Due in large part to the work of the German psychiatrist Emil Kraepelin (1856–1926), delusions were increasingly seen as a key symptom of schizophrenia and related diagnoses. (Kraepelin founded the Department of Psychiatry at the University of Munich. Alois Alzheimer studied with him while investigating the dementia that came to bear his name.) And that put delusions on the wrong side of a line that psychiatrists were drawing between so-called neurotic illnesses, such as depression and anxiety, and psychotic disorders like schizophrenia. Neuroses were deemed to be the psychological product of life events. Psychoses, on the other hand, were viewed as the result of biological illnesses. In 1913 Karl Jaspers' (1883–1969) landmark *General Psychopathology* noted:

> The most profound distinction in psychic life seems to be that between what is meaningful and allows empathy [i.e. neurosis] and what in its particular way is ununderstandable, mad in the literal sense [psychosis] . . .

Paranoid delusions were dismissed as so much empty verbiage: nonsense from a damaged or decayed brain. (Kraepelin, for example, saw schizophrenia – or what he called 'dementia praecox' – as a neurodegenerative disease. There could be, he believed, no cure.) The idea of listening to someone describe their suspicious thoughts, as I and so many other clinicians do almost every working day, would no doubt have struck our predecessors as preposterous. As late as 1969, the third edition of the influential textbook *Clinical Psychiatry* was advising mental health professionals that:

Although it is a waste of time to argue with a paranoid patient about his delusions, he may still be persuaded to keep them to himself, to repress them as far as possible and to forgo the aggressive action they might suggest, in general to conduct his life as if they did not exist.

Indeed, not talking about delusions was regarded as potentially therapeutic. Reward people for not expressing their fears, psychologists reasoned, and they'd eventually stop thinking about them too. This technique was known as 'token economy' and it was widespread in the 1970s. In one clinical trial in Vermont, for example, patients in a ward for 'paranoid schizophrenics' were given tokens for 'talking correctly'. These tokens could be exchanged for items including 'meals, extra dessert, visits to the canteen, cigarettes, time off the ward, time in the TV and game room, time in bedroom between 8 a.m. and 9 p.m., visitors, books and magazines, recreation, dances on other wards'. It didn't work. Most patients modified their behaviour temporarily: doubtless they quickly figured out how to play the system. But 'changes in a patient's delusional system and general mental status could not be detected by a psychiatrist'.

The idea that paranoia was merely a symptom of a condition like schizophrenia remained dominant when I started out as a clinical psychologist – which explains why there was so little interest in it among professionals. The legacy of Heinroth and Bleuler was still influential too: 'paranoia' was used to describe a type of psychosis principally characterised by delusions of all types. It was this condition – known today as delusional disorder – that the *Oxford Companion to the Mind* was describing in 1987: 'True paranoia is, fortunately, rare; it has a bad prognosis and is not amenable to any known treatment.' In fact, clinicians and researchers continued to use the term 'paranoia' to denote delusions in general – regardless of whether they appeared in the context of schizophrenia, delusional disorder, or some other diagnosis. It's not gone away. A few years ago a letter to the *British Journal of Psychiatry* scolded me for describing paranoia as the unfounded fear that others intend to cause you harm: 'the correct meaning of "paranoid" is "delusional"'. And though those delusions might include 'persecutory' thoughts, when I began thinking seriously about the issue there was no agreed definition of what exactly made a delusion persecutory. You could find at least three variants in psychiatric textbooks, and all were slightly different. In fact, the term was used so loosely that I decided to write a paper to define it. Not everyone felt this was a worthwhile undertaking. One reviewer likened it to the medieval theological debate about the number of angels who could dance upon a pinhead. But precision has always seemed to me to be essential. How can scientific knowledge advance if we don't agree on what it is we're talking about? How can we develop effective therapies unless we specify the nature of the problem?

So, what kind of content typifies persecutory delusions? They comprise dire fears about intentional harm – now or in the future – at the hands of others. As such, they constitute the sharpest end of the spectrum of mistrust. That imagined harm can take all manner of forms. For a relatively small number of people the threat is existential: their very life is in danger from malign conspiratorial forces. But although dramatic cases like James Tilly Matthews have attracted most attention, they are exceptional. Most of the people I see are concerned about far more prosaic problems: being excluded and ridiculed; deliberately wound up by nasty neighbours; smeared as a paedophile; getting roughed up by local youths; or being singled out as a target for burglary or vandalism. When we look at paranoia in the general population, a similar picture emerges. Highly implausible beliefs are rare. Workaday worries about friends, colleagues and acquaintances are common.

So much for names and definitions. If we discount the idea that paranoia is random babble produced by cerebral injury or illness, what were the initial psychological accounts?

Paranoia as protection

'The purpose of paranoia is to ward off an idea that is incompatible with the ego, by projecting its substance into the external world.'

Sigmund Freud

For almost a hundred years, Western psychiatry was dominated by the ideas of Sigmund Freud. For the psychoanalyst Anthony Storr, Freudian 'psychoanalysis has become the dominant idiom for the discussion of the human personality and of human relations'. So, what did Freud have to say about paranoia? In an article written in 1915, he relates the story of a thirty-year-old woman, 'a most attractive and handsome girl', who had become close to 'a highly cultivated and attractive man' from her work-place. There was, apparently, no question of marriage. But the man 'had pleaded that it was senseless to sacrifice to social convention all that they both longed for and had an indisputable right to enjoy, some thing that could enrich their life as nothing else could'. Persuaded of the man's discretion, the woman had agreed to visit her lover's apartment.

While they were making love on her second visit, the woman was startled by a knock or click from the direction of a writing desk that stood near the window. Her lover assured her that the noise had been produced by a clock sitting on the desk. However:

As she was leaving the house she had met two men on the staircase, who whispered something to each other when they saw her. One of the strangers was carrying something which was wrapped up and looked like a small box. She was much exercised over this meeting, and on her way home she had already put together the following notions: the box might easily have been a camera, and the man a photographer who had been hidden behind the curtain while she was in the room; the click had been the noise of the shutter; the photograph had been taken as soon as he saw her in a particularly compromising position . . .

The incident didn't do much for the relationship: 'From that moment nothing could abate her suspicion of her lover. She pursued him with reproaches and pestered him for explanations and reassurances, not only when they met but also by letter. But it was in vain that he tried to convince her that his feelings were sincere and that her suspicions were entirely without foundation.'

Freud and the woman met twice for consultations. He concluded that there had been no noise from a clock, a camera, or indeed anything else. The meeting with the men on the stairs had been entirely fortuitous. Why then should the woman believe that her lover had arranged for her to be photographed, and thus potentially ruined? Freud argued that the idea was defensive: 'the patient protected herself against her love for a man by means of a paranoia delusion'. But why should she want protection? What underlying purpose did her paranoia serve? According to Freud, a battle had been raging in the woman's unconscious mind. She was torn between her 'homosexual attachment' to her mother and her desire to escape from that attachment. By accepting her lover's advances, she struck a blow against the dependence on her mother. But the latter had proven too strong:

'by making ingenious use of some accidental circumstances [her paranoid delusion] destroyed this love and thus successfully carried through the purpose of the mother-complex.'

In Freud's view this was not a one-off:

> Distrusting my own experience on the subject, I have during the last few years joined with my friends C. G. Jung of Zurich and Sándor Ferenczi of Budapest in investigating upon this single point a number of cases of paranoid disorder which have come under observation. The patients whose histories provided the material for this enquiry included both men and women, and varied in race, occupation, and social standing. Yet we were astonished to find that in all of these cases a defence against a homosexual wish was clearly recognisable at the very centre of the conflict which underlay the disease, and that it was in an attempt to master an unconsciously reinforced current of homosexuality that they had all of them come to grief.

What are we to make of this theory today? It's true that Freud, unlike many twentieth-century psychiatrists, was profoundly interested in his patients' paranoid thoughts. He regarded them as statements that were abundant in meaning rather than empty of it. Yet, though scientists have looked for evidence to support Freud's model of paranoia, they've not found it. Indeed, one 1975 review of the hotchpotch of studies undertaken to date concluded that patients with persecutory delusions were *more likely* to report homosexual thoughts. As it happens, though, the idea that paranoia functions as a defence was to re-emerge in the 1990s. This time it came from clinical psychologists rather than psychoanalysts. They argued that paranoia functioned as protection not against homosexual desire but against negative views of the self. But though the putative threat was different, the mechanism was similar: to minimise internal psychological distress, we subconsciously externalise our emotions. The pain of low self-esteem is masked by our fear of other people. *It's not me: it's you.*

From air looms to aeroplanes

The theory that paranoia is a defence against deeply buried fears has never convinced me. I think it's far more about conscious thoughts than some Freudian unconscious. And in this, and much more besides, my ideas align with those of another hugely influential doctor: Aaron Beck.

Beck, who died in 2021 at the age of 100, was the founder of cognitive behaviour therapy and without question the most significant psychiatrist of the last century. He was also a mentor to me since the day in late 1998 when an email from him appeared in my inbox. Naturally I assumed the email had been sent in error. At the time I was a trainee on the clinical psychology doctoral course at the Institute of Psychiatry. How could Beck know my name? That he should invite me to Philadelphia for a meeting of cognitive psychologists working on psychosis beggared belief. Sheepishly, I explained that while I would have been delighted to attend, I had no funds for the trip. No problem, he replied with characteristic generosity, we'll cover your expenses. It was a fantastic experience. With Beck covering my air fare, on my way back I was able to make my first visit to New York. And I can still fit into the Penn State T-shirt I bought from the university bookstore. But the week had a slightly nerve-wracking beginning. On the first evening, the group were due to meet at 6 p.m. at a sports bar in down-town Philadelphia. I was on time. But as I entered the bar, I realised with horror that the only other person there was Beck himself. I needn't have worried. Beck had a special talent for making you feel that you were exactly the person he wanted to be talking to. These gatherings of cognitive psychologists – which I named, much to his embarrassment, Beckfest – have continued every year to this day.

In the 1950s Beck trained in Freudian psychotherapy at the Philadelphia Psychoanalytic Institute, but he was never entirely at ease in the role: 'The idea was that if you sat back and listened and said "Ah-hah," somehow secrets would come out. And you would get exhausted just from the helplessness of it.' Beck recalled the moment that he decided to change course. Listening to a female patient describe her sexual liaisons, he asked her: 'How does talking about this make you feel?' 'I feel anxious,' the woman replied. 'You are anxious because you are having to confront some of your sexual desires,' Beck said. 'And you are anxious because you expect me to be disapproving of these desires.' 'Actually, Dr Beck,' the woman explained, 'I'm afraid that I'm boring you.'

Beck taught us that the explanation – and resolution – for psychological problems typically lies not in unconscious 'secrets', but in conscious thoughts: what you think determines what you feel. So there's no need for a therapist to try to excavate long-buried desires and memories. Better instead to be attentive to what the patient tells you about their thoughts, feelings and experiences. In his Freudian incarnation, Beck once investigated the theory that people were depressed because of a masochistic desire to feel pain. But there were no hidden motives. 'They saw themselves as losers because that's the way they saw themselves.'

I think the same is true of paranoia. Paranoia isn't a defence against repressed homosexual desire or subconscious low self-esteem. On the contrary, it is rooted in, and fuelled by, a sense of personal vulnerability. And this vulnerability isn't hidden away in the depths of the unconscious. To find it, we just have to listen to what our patients tell us. As Beck noted: 'There is more on the surface than meets the eye.' And indeed people susceptible to paranoia are much more likely to endorse statements like these: *I am unloved. I am worthless. I am weak. I am vulnerable. I am bad. I am a failure.* They are also likely to believe that: *Other people are hostile. Other people are harsh. Other people are unforgiving. Other people are bad. Other people are devious. Other people are nasty.* This shouldn't come as a surprise. After all, if you see yourself as weak and worthless, and other people as strong and cruel, fear seems a rational response. As we'll see in the next chapter, that fear isn't confined to people with psychosis. In fact, there are signs that it may be increasingly widespread.

4.

The virtual tube

'I think they're trying to frame me.'

As with many British psychiatric hospitals in the early 2000s (and still, sadly, today), the waiting room when I worked at the Maudsley resembled an unloved Portakabin: a large rectangular box housing several dozen plastic chairs, a water cooler, and almost nothing else. Set into one wall was a hatch, to which patients were called to collect their prescriptions. The place smelled strongly of stale cigarettes. By way of decoration, a few paintings by patients had been hung on the walls. But the battle had been lost. Nothing, it seems, could overcome the ambience of neglect. Many of the staff were brilliant. But, looking at the room, who would have believed that this was a place where unhappy people came to feel better?

Today I lead Mr Gayle through a set of security doors and head up the stairs to the third floor. I no longer take patients in the tiny lift. Being surrounded by other people with no easy means of escape is a typical trigger for paranoid thoughts. Even worse, a few years ago the elevator juddered to an unscheduled halt between floors. Jammed inside like passengers on a rush-hour commuter train were four people, including myself and a patient feeling acutely paranoid who believed the NHS had deliberately engineered the problem to upset him. We were stuck for just a minute or two, but it was long enough for me to resolve never to risk a repetition.

The consulting rooms in the Maudsley at that time were no more inviting than the waiting room downstairs. Typically, they contained only an old desk and a couple of chairs, one behind the desk and a slightly less comfortable one in front of it. But I swiftly learned to be thankful to have any room, however bleakly impersonal, in which to meet patients. To obtain one, processes had to be followed. One of those processes was administrative. You entered the details in the ledger held by the receptionists downstairs. The other, much more important process was diplomatic. You did whatever it took to remain on friendly terms with the receptionists. This was no hardship, but it could not be left to chance. Therapists all knew what it was like to comb the corridors with a patient in tow, desperately opening door after door in the hope of finding a vacant room. Canny clinicians booked far in advance. The pool shrank at an extraordinary rate. Securing a room always felt like a victory.

'Do you have any idea who may want to frame you?'

Kieran Gayle is smiling hesitantly, but I know how debilitating his paranoia can be. Indeed, that is why he is sitting with me now. Problems began for him ten years ago, just as he was about to start his second year of university. (This is common: psychosis often begins in young adulthood.) He'd been dealing with a lot of stress at the time – worrying about his academic work, struggling to sort out accommodation with friends, and getting on badly with his girlfriend. Before university his self-confidence had been high; that things had apparently fallen apart so swiftly had been 'utterly demoralising'. He'd become anxious and depressed. He came to believe that he had religious powers and that, as a result, people in league with the devil were spying on him. He could tell who was doing this by looking at their eyes: the pupils were abnormally large or small. Over the years, medication has brought some improvement for Mr Gayle. But the paranoia has still been causing him problems and so, eventually, he has been referred to our specialist clinic. He is thirty years old but looks younger. He wears faded jeans and brightly polished black shoes.

He shrugs. 'I don't know. Someone powerful. The police, maybe. They use bugs to listen in on me. All my thoughts. My bad thoughts. Maybe I want to hit someone. Or steal something.' He looks at me sheepishly. 'It sounds ridiculous. I know they're delusions. Usually I don't believe them much. But sometimes they feel totally real.'

'What do you think these people mean to do?' I ask.

He pauses. Sighs. 'It's embarrassing talking about it.' Another pause. Then a deep intake of breath, a metaphorical run-up before the words tumble out in a rush: 'To get me sent to prison. Then they'll torture me. They'll kill me.' He sinks back in his chair. 'I'm easy meat. Anyone can make a fool out of me. They know that. It's just the way I am.'

'You haven't ended up in prison. Why do you think that is?'

'I'm on my guard. They know I'm alert to what they're doing. So they bide their time.'

'And what makes you think people are spying on you? What do you notice?'

'It's just a feeling. I haven't seen anyone doing it. But then I guess I wouldn't. They aren't amateurs.'

'Can you describe that feeling to me?'

'Um,' Mr Gayle runs his fingers through his hair, scratches his scalp. 'Sometimes it's just like a heightened awareness of myself – my body, my thoughts, where I am, that sort of thing. I feel a bit anxious. Other times it's more extreme. My head fills up with thoughts – they race around my brain.' Mr Gayle looks at the floor. 'It feels,' he says, 'like I'm losing control.'

I saw Mr Gayle every week for the next nine months.

Not so rare after all?

Like Mr Gayle, most people diagnosed with schizophrenia experience persecutory delusions. Around 50 per cent also hear threatening voices. In the UK around seven people in every thousand experience a schizophrenia-like disorder each year. Globally, it has been estimated that 24 million people are affected. But the fact that we have these figures shouldn't be taken for granted: measuring the prevalence of psychological disorders is a relatively novel development. For a long time, the only data available were hospital admissions. Even then, there wasn't much consistency in diagnosis. With no standard classificatory system for mental health conditions, clinicians had a lot of latitude when it came to interpreting their patients' symptoms. They might easily disagree not only on the nature of an individual's problem, but also on whether the patient had a problem at all. As David Barlow and V. Mark Durand have noted: 'As late as 1959 there were at least nine different systems of varying usefulness for classifying psychological disorders worldwide.' Things really began to change in the 1980s with the general adoption of two landmark texts: the American Psychiatric Association's *Diagnostic and Statistical Manual of Mental Disorders* (DSM) and the World Health Organization's *International Classification of Diseases and Health Related Problems* (ICD). As the two have evolved, their approach has been coordinated. Mental health professionals are increasingly able to sing from the same hymn sheet.

With standardised diagnosis, standardised research suddenly became feasible. In the late 1980s, for example, no one knew how prevalent psychological disorders were in the vast mass of people who never came to the clinic. Now it was possible to find out. For the first time, questions normally asked of patients with schizophrenia in psychiatric hospitals were put to the rest of the population. The results of these early efforts sometimes surprised their authors. Using data from the National Institute of Mental Health Epidemiologic Catchment Area Program, Allen Tien and William Eaton analysed rates of psychosis in more than fifteen thousand people from five US cities:

> Rates for schizophrenia from registry data [i.e. hospital admission] may be underestimates. . . . the ECA Program appears to have detected the incidence of a syndrome that resembles clinical schizophrenia, in terms of sociodemographic pattern, with an estimated incidence rate of 0.2 cases per 100 people per year, much higher than estimates from any registry-based studies.

Given what we know about schizophrenia, we can be pretty sure that many of the people picked up by the ECA survey were experiencing persecutory thoughts. But what about the overwhelming majority of the general public who *didn't* meet the criteria for a schizophrenia diagnosis – or indeed for any psychological disorder? Did they ever experience paranoia? We had little idea. There were hardly any data. In 2004 I began with a rough and ready internet survey of twelve hundred students. (The Institute of Psychiatry had become affiliated to King's College London a few years previously; in those days it was easy to email the entire university.) I was very surprised to discover that around a third of the participants were regularly troubled by paranoid thoughts. At least once a week – and in many cases much more often – over 50 per cent felt that they needed to be on their guard against other people. Forty-two per cent thought that people might be making negative remarks about them. Forty-eight per cent believed that strangers and friends alike had looked at them critically. And 34 per cent worried that people were laughing at them.

Of course, an online survey of self-selected participants, all of a similar age, isn't ideal. But in this case, it turned out to be a reasonably accurate guide. Subsequently, study after study reinforced the idea that paranoia was far more common than anyone had suspected. Take the nationally representative 2007 Adult Psychiatric Morbidity Survey (APMS) in England. The aim of the APMS is 'to collect data on mental health among adults aged 16 and over living in private households in England'. Its range is intentionally broad: the idea is to gauge 'the prevalence of both treated and untreated psychiatric disorders'. Delving into the multitude of assessment questions, I was excited to unearth some that bore directly on paranoia. Of the more than seven thousand adults interviewed, I found that 18.6 per cent had thought at some point in the previous twelve months that people were against them. Eight per cent believed that people had deliberately acted to harm them. Almost 2 per cent had felt that groups were plotting to cause them serious harm. In another representative survey of 8,580 UK adults that asked people to reflect on their experiences over the previous twelve months, 21 per cent reported that they'd sometimes felt that people were hostile towards them; 9 per cent had suspected that their thoughts were being manipulated; and 1.5 per cent had feared a conspiracy to cause them serious harm. A survey of 1,005 adults registered at a GP practice in Manhattan found that 10.6 per cent had at some time in their life thought they were being followed or spied upon. Almost 7 per cent had believed they were the victims of a plot. Around 5 per cent had suspected that they were either being secretly tested or experimented upon. All in all, the likely scale of paranoia in the community was remarkable.

The fact that mistrust is widespread among people who have never been diagnosed with a psychological problem, let alone spent time on a psychiatric ward, doesn't only tell us something about paranoia. It speaks to a radically different conception of mental health in general. In light of data like these, the idea that paranoia is confined to the small percentage of people with schizophrenia is no longer tenable. We are social creatures. We live in an extraordinarily intricate, diverse and dynamic web of relationships with other people. The friend in whom we confide how we are feeling. The taxi driver who ferries us home after a night out. The waiter to whom we hand over our credit card. Choice after choice after choice. An infinity of forks in the road. We seldom reflect upon it, but our days comprise a succession of decisions as to whether to trust other people or not. And because we seldom know what another person is thinking, it's easy to misread intentions. From this perspective, paranoia isn't necessarily a symptom of illness. Rather, it's a marker on a continuum of experience. At opposite ends of that continuum are the few people who never experience paranoia and those with profoundly troubling and enduring delusions. Most of us lie somewhere in between, though our precise location may vary over time. In this sense, mistrust is no different to happiness, sadness, worry, self-confidence or fearfulness. Indeed, it's just like mental health in general. There is no hard and fast dividing line between mental health and mental illness. It's not a binary proposition: *I am mentally well/I am mentally ill*. Better instead to think of gradations and nuances, and of people travelling backwards and forwards along that continuum as they progress through their lives.

Despite the welter of figures I've just presented, it's true that gauging paranoia can be tricky. After all, how do we judge whether a reported threat is real or not? Maybe the survey data tells us less about the prevalence of imaginary fears than it does about how perilous life can be? Maybe some of the respondents were right to suspect that people were being hostile towards them? Take the patient who tells me that a man deliberately elbowed her into a busy road while she was out shopping. I have no means of knowing whether her account is accurate or a paranoid interpretation of an inadvertent mishap. Even if I'd seen the incident, I couldn't be sure that the other person had purposely pushed her off the pavement. (For that reason, I always keep an open mind. Therapeutically, my focus is on the future and much less on what may or may not have happened in the past.)

But we do have ways to corroborate these sorts of data. And it turns out that the picture they paint is accurate. In the survey of ten thousand UK adults I commissioned in 2023, 40 per cent said they felt more fearful of other people than they should do. A similar number reported exaggerated fears that others might try to embarrass them. And when we asked whether they would like help to trust other people, 38 per cent answered maybe and 17 per cent responded yes. Note that these people aren't reporting hostility from others. They aren't claiming that they've been victimised in some way. We don't have to wonder whether they are simply reporting actual harm. On the contrary: they are telling us just how mistrustful they have become. Crucially, these responses correlate closely with the answers to paranoia questionnaires. The people who say they're afraid of harm at the hands of others are also likely to acknowledge that their anxiety is exaggerated. In other words, what people are reporting in paranoia assessments isn't actual threat: it's unwarranted mistrust.

So, we can tell a lot by cross-referencing various types of survey data. But to complement what people were telling me, what I really wanted was an *experimental test* of paranoia. If I could expose a large group of people to the same benign experience, I could see how many reacted in a mistrustful way. I could then begin to investigate why they behaved as they did.

Because if I could ensure the environment was threat-free, I could be certain that the explanation lay not in the experience but rather in the minds of the participants. But how would one devise such an experiment? The answer to that conundrum came with a chance visit to the cave.

Into the cave

'VR is one of the scientific, philosophical, and techno-logical frontiers of our era. It is a means for creating comprehensive illusions that you're in a different place, perhaps a fantastical, alien environment, perhaps with a body that is far from human. And yet it is also the farthest-reaching apparatus for researching what a human being is in the terms of cognition and perception.'
Jaron Lanier, *Dawn of the New Everything* (2017)

Today I have headed across the Thames, swapping scruffy and suburban south London for the Georgian splendour of Bloomsbury. It is 2001 and I am embarking on my own space odyssey. Deep in the bowels of University College London (UCL), I make my rather tentative way to the computer science department for a demonstration by Professor Mel Slater. Mel, I have been informed, is a pioneer of something called virtual reality. Mel appeared recently on BBC Radio 4, where he caught the imagination of my colleagues Paul Bebbington and Elizabeth Kuipers. Enterprisingly, Paul and Elizabeth have set up today's demo. In the months and years to come I will have a front-row seat for Mel's brilliant psychological experiments in VR. Right now, however, I have only the sketchiest sense of what to expect. I am along for the ride.

To reach UCL's computer science department, we thread through corridor after corridor. On the way we pass a friendly-looking gentleman wearing a large hat and antiquated clothes, and holding a walking stick. He is sitting on a chair in a large, glass-fronted wooden case. It is the philosopher Jeremy Bentham, or rather his 'auto-icon', fashioned from his skeleton and a waxen replica of his head. Bentham always intended that his actual head be used, and is said to have kept in his pocket the pair of glass eyes that would gaze out from it. But the mummification of the head was not a success. It was deemed too ghastly to display, and a wax version was substituted. Bentham had stipulated in his will that his corpse be donated to his friend, the surgeon Thomas Southwood Smith. He suggested it 'be used as the means of illustrating a series of lectures to which scientific & literary men are to be invited'. This was a political act by Bentham: until the year of his death, 1832, it had been illegal to leave one's body for medical research. The auto-icon, designed by Bentham himself, is what remains after the cadaver's dissection by Southwood Smith, who gifted the figure to UCL in 1850.

We have reached our destination. The contrast between Bentham's ancient simulacrum and what goes on here in the lab of UCL's Professor of Virtual Environments could not be starker.

In 1962 a young PhD student at the Massachusetts Institute of Technology named Ivan Sutherland invented the Sketchpad. It allowed people to manipulate images on a computer screen using a light pen. This was revolutionary. Sutherland had built the first graphical user interface. Suddenly it was possible for humans to interact with a computer via a screen instead of the laboriously programmed punched cards and magnetic tape reels that had been the norm. As fellow VR pioneer Jaron Lanier has written: 'The impact was spectacular. It's often called the best computer demo of all time.' But Sutherland was merely warming up. In 1969 he built a headset through which the wearer could see what Sutherland described as 'virtual worlds'.

Sutherland's headset has come to be known as the Sword of Damocles. (In fact, the name originally denoted the overhead beam from which the headset was suspended: no user could bear its weight unsupported.) The hulking tech was by today's standards rudimentary in computing power, but it included what are still the essential components of VR. A computer generated an image, a display system presented the sensory information, and a tracker fed back the user's position and orientation to update the image. For the user, data from the natural world was superseded by information about an imaginary world that changed in response to their actions. Backed by the financial muscle of companies like Meta and Sony, virtual reality today is a poster child for the consumer electronics market. It is arguably the shiniest new toy in gaming technology. Weighing just 500 grams, headsets are far lighter and immeasurably more comfortable than Sutherland's prototype. The immersive experience they deliver is breathtakingly sophisticated, light years away from the floating hollow cube with which Sutherland began. But the technical model is essentially the same. For all the marketing hullabaloo, in these fundamentals not much has really changed in VR.

It is almost impossible to convey just how extraordinary virtual reality can be. It is often said that writing about music is like dancing about architecture, and I think the same is true for verbal descriptions of VR. To understand its power, you really need to strap on a headset. One of the many surprising things about VR is that, although you know the scenarios aren't real, your mind and body behave as if they were. Stand on a virtual ledge several hundred metres above the city streets, for example, and you instinctively recoil. There is nothing artificial about the fear the experience induces. For psychologists this emotional fidelity unlocks a myriad of exciting possibilities for understanding how the mind works and, as we'll see in Chapter 13, for treating mental health problems. But I didn't know that then.

Mel Slater's VR lab was a large, subterranean, windowless room with black walls and thick, light-absorbent curtains. In the centre was a cuboid space in which the magic took place. This was the CAVE Automatic Virtual Environment, its name inspired by a passage from Plato's *Republic* in which the philosopher learns about reality from images on a cave wall. In the VR Cave, an image is projected onto three walls and the floor. Wearing stereoscopic glasses, the user can walk through the virtual environment, using a joystick to move in their chosen direction.

'Your turn,' smiled Mel, proffering the glasses and joystick. 'Oh, and you'll need to take off your shoes.' A little nervously, and conscious of the rather large hole in my sock, I took my place within the walls of the CAVE and waited for . . . I wasn't quite sure what. Suddenly I found myself in a large, bright, parquet-floored library. Tentatively at first, and then with increasing confidence, I explored my new surroundings. Towards me walked a young man in a boxy blue suit, oddly rectangular black shoes and a vivid red tie. VR characters, Mel explained, were termed 'avatars'. Later I visited a virtual pub where I was confronted by a belligerent Arsenal fan. (This was the prototype for a fascinating experiment in social psychology involving forty real-life Arsenal supporters. Mel was investigating whether bystanders are more likely to offer help if they identify with a stranger, in this case because of the football team they support. In a nutshell: they are.) The sensation was curious. There was no mistaking the computer-generated nature of the scenes. Nevertheless, I felt that I had been somewhere new and that I had experienced something meaningful. This was much more than some trick of the light.

The tech was cool, for sure. I'd never experienced anything like it. And as a psychologist I was intrigued by the way in which VR allowed one to create and control social situations. But as I handed the glasses and joystick back to Mel, I wondered whether those situations would trigger sufficiently realistic responses. (Being watched by Mel, Paul and Elizabeth hadn't helped my own sense of immersion.) Would users see the computer characters – the avatars – as beings with thoughts, intentions and feelings? If they did, I suddenly realised, we might have a way to achieve the impossible: to observe paranoia in a laboratory setting.

There was only one way to find out. We designed an experiment using a modified version of Mel's virtual library space. Shelves lined the walls. Computer-generated students sat at two reading desks, positioned so that some of the characters would always be behind the user. Occasionally, these avatars would smile, look up, or talk to one another. Crucially, we programmed them to seem pleasant, or at the very least neutral. If our participants reported hostility from the characters, we'd know it was paranoia. For this pilot study we recruited twenty-four students from UCL, most of them computer scientists. (We had no funding for the study so had to keep things simple – and cheap.) Their task was straightforward: 'Please explore the room, and try to form some impression of what you think about the people in the room and what they think about you.' Each of the participants spent five minutes in our VR library. As we expected, most enjoyed the experience, finding the avatars friendly and welcoming. But a minority of the participants perceived the characters as threatening:

'They were very ignorant and unfriendly. Sometimes appeared hostile, sometimes rude. It was their space: you're the stranger.'

'They were telling me to go away.'

'One person was very shy and another had hated me. The two women looked more threatening.'

'Some were intimidating.'

Nine of the twenty-four volunteers said that someone in the room had it in for them. Thirteen thought that the characters might be talking about them behind their back. And these individuals were also more likely to report suspicious thoughts in the outside world. As I interviewed our participants after their trip to the virtual library, the penny dropped. I began to grasp just how powerful a medium VR could be. It was so compelling that users would attribute thoughts to patently computer-generated characters and respond emotionally as if those characters were real. Visually, our virtual library and the avatars within it were pretty rough and ready – certainly a very long way from any kind of photo-realism. That they could provoke such a range of responses was astounding. Those responses, moreover, were a perfect demonstration of the way in which we all subjectively construct our interpretation of events. You can give everyone the same experience, but you can't assume you'll get the same reaction. Now I saw the immense potential that VR offered clinical psychology. Now I was a believer. It was time to step things up. I applied for, and was awarded, a Wellcome Trust Fellowship. The objective: to use VR to learn about paranoia.

The virtual tube

In the summer of 2006 Kat Pugh and I enlisted one hundred men and one hundred women from the area around King's College London to take part in what we advertised as a study of 'people's reactions in virtual reality'. (Over the years I have been fortunate to recruit an extraordinarily talented group of psychology assistants. Kat was the first.) In fact, the study was the first large-scale VR investigation of paranoia. Anyone with a history of schizophrenia or another severe psychological disorder – and therefore a potentially elevated vulnerability to paranoia – was excluded. In other respects, the group was representative of the local adult population.

Participants were invited to my new VR lab at King's, a medium-sized room with cushions lining the walls: it is easy to lose track of where you are when you're wearing a headset. Proudly, we showed our participants how to put on our state-of-the-art VR headset. State-of-the-art for 2006, that is. Unlike today's VR, for which all you need is a headset and a pair of hand controllers, the Virtual Research VR1280 headset was tethered by cable to a high-powered computer. Meanwhile, the user's movements were tracked not by cameras built into the headset (standard practice today) but by a constellation of sensors embedded in the ceiling. The study would have been impossible without the support of the Wellcome Trust. The VR equipment alone cost over £45,000. Even more importantly, we needed to recruit a VR computer scientist. Mel came up trumps again, pointing us in the direction of Angus Antley, one of his protégés. Angus programmed the VR software and looked after the hardware, all of which required considerable expertise. Today one could achieve the same immersive experience – indeed probably far better – on a headset costing just a few hundred pounds. And you wouldn't need to worry about the unseen tangle of wires connecting you to the computer: a trip hazard if ever there were one. Tethered VR always seems to necessitate an awkward little dance as the user and the person overseeing the session attempt to avoid tripping over the snaking coils of cable.

For our VR scenario, we chose a situation with which virtually all our participants were likely to be familiar: a ride on the

London Underground. It was a scenario rich in the social inter-action on which paranoia thrives. And like the lift at the Maudsley, it could also make you feel cramped or trapped – again, a trigger for paranoia. (By no coincidence, the VR scenario we designed next was an elevator.) The London Underground is used by around two million people every day. With its 270 stations and 250 miles of track, and more than five hundred trains operating at rush hour, it is one of the world's busiest metro systems. Our partici-pants experienced a small sample of the hurly-burly, taking a four-minute ride in VR between two stops on the Victoria line. With them in the virtual carriage were several computer-generated passengers. As in our previous experiment, we programmed these passengers to be neutral in their behaviour. If a participant looked at the avatars for any length of time, some would respond by looking in their direction and one would occasionally smile. But we did our best to ensure that none appeared at all hostile.

After they'd removed their headsets, we asked the participants what they had made of their fellow passengers. Many people found the avatars unremarkable:

'Felt like a normal tube. People just trying to get where they want to go.'

'Didn't think anyone thought anything about me. All getting on with own business. Nobody seemed to notice me.'

'I thought they were like people on the tube – some smile, others ignore you. I thought everyone kept themselves to themselves.'

This was no surprise. It was precisely how the avatars had been programmed to appear. Other participants found them rather more appealing:

'It was nice, much nicer than a real experience – people aren't so forthcoming with their feelings in a real situation. Thought they were pretty friendly.'

'People were generally very friendly.'

'One guy was checking me out – flattering.'

'There were people smiling at you, which was nice.'

'The man in the pink jumper might have chatted me up.'

For a sizeable minority of participants, however, their fellow passengers seemed neither neutral nor friendly. Instead, they appeared unpleasant and threatening:

'Thought a couple of the men were stuck up and nasty. Lady sitting down laughed at me when I walked past.'

'There was an aggressive person – his intention was to intimidate me and make me feel uneasy.'

'One guy looked pissed off and maybe one guy flicked the finger at me.'

'There was a man who tried to stare me out. But I didn't give him any ammunition. Believe his intention was to start an argument.'

'There's something dodgy about one guy. Like he was about to do something – assault someone, plant a bomb, say something not nice to me, be aggressive.'

Every one of the two hundred participants saw and heard the same thing. Yet their responses were extraordinarily varied. Clearly, how we react to a situation is determined by our *interpretation* of events: we construct our world and its meaning. But interpreting other people's behaviour is an awkward business. We have no reliable way of judging intention. We can only guess, based on what we see and on our previous experience, at what other people are thinking and feeling. It is very easy to get things wrong.

The results of our experiment were covered in the *Sun*, which was a novelty. 'Third of Brits are paranoid (Don't worry, we're not talking about you)', the newspaper announced. Our virtual tube ride had indeed triggered paranoid thoughts in a third of our participants. We knew that the avatars had done nothing to warrant this reaction, because we had deliberately programmed them not to. What this shows is just how ubiquitous mistrust is. For a great many of us, suspicion seems to be the default setting. We are hypersensitive to threat, constantly vigilant in anticipation of harm. We feel embattled.

But perhaps there was something special about our VR scenario? Maybe people would have reacted differently in an actual tube carriage? It is unlikely. Decades of research have shown that people behave in VR much as they would in real life. To be certain, we compared the reactions of individuals who reported paranoia in everyday life and those who did not. Sure enough, the former were much more likely to experience persecutory thoughts in VR.

I wanted to know if there was anything else distinctive about the people who experienced paranoid thoughts in our experiment. To find out, before their VR experience we asked the participants to complete ninety minutes' worth of psychological assessments. Those who were prone to paranoia turned out to be also more susceptible to anxiety and depression. They were worriers. They scored highly for what is known in the jargon as interpersonal sensitivity: feelings of inadequacy and inferiority, particularly in comparison with others and, as such, a tendency to regard themselves as a soft target. Their self-esteem was low. And they were much more likely to think negatively about other people – for example, to believe that they are devious, unforgiving or nasty. They tended to be less flexible in their thinking, less able or willing to consider options and adapt to situations. They were more likely to experience what psychologists call 'perceptual anomalies': being highly sensitive to sound, light or smells, for instance; experiencing strange bodily sensations; or hearing and seeing things that other people don't. And their family relationships were often problematic. The results marked a big step forward in the effort to understand paranoia. They were crucial components in the psychological model I was gradually putting together. Now we had a definition of paranoia, and the means to measure it both in the laboratory and at scale in the community, it was time to press on at full speed to understand the causes.

5.

People can't be trusted

'The 2015 Paris attacks are not my story: I didn't lose a loved one, didn't see anyone shot dead in front of me. But suffice to say that those hours I spent trapped in a bar near the Bataclan not knowing if they were coming for us, convinced they were coming for us, prodded my condition awake once more.

This is how I become, essentially, agoraphobic: I stop taking public transport. I fly once, and spend the descent lying in the aisle being given oxygen. I rarely go to restaurants and bars (when I do go, I sit away from the window, and am jumpy and distracted). I do not go to shopping malls, cinemas, railway stations or squares. I do go to work – I take a taxi there and back, and spend the entire time in the newspaper's office wondering when they are coming to kill us. Sometimes, the fire alarm goes off and I walk out of the building with my whole body shaking and go home, where I sob, and then sleep for hours. I am lucky: my editor is very understanding.

Other things that frighten me: people on mopeds. Cars that are parked with people in them. Suitcases that appear to have no owner, people wearing bulky coats. I look up at planes overhead and am convinced they will drop from *the sky. On Christmas Day, a low-flying helicopter reduces me to such paralysing terror that I lock myself in the bathroom.'*

The writer Rhiannon Lucy Cosslett was violently assaulted in 2010. In the aftermath, she became terrified that someone, somewhere would finish the job her assailant had begun. Ceaselessly on edge, Cosslett was wracked by nightmares and buffeted by graphic flashbacks. Trauma-focused CBT helped Cosslett to recover. But in the wake of the Paris terrorist attacks of November 2015, in which 130 people were killed and over 400 injured, she came to believe that 'the world is conspiring to kill me'. There was no respite from the fear: 'I feel as though I'm about to die almost every waking moment.'

Paranoia and trauma

Sadly, Rhiannon Lucy Cosslett's story is all too common. Almost a third of adults in England report having experienced at least one traumatic incident – that is, an event putting them, or someone close to them, at risk of serious harm or death. For some people, those experiences result in post-traumatic stress disorder. In PTSD the fear that helps us survive dangerous situations (the famous 'fight or flight' response) continues long after that situation is over. The alarm keeps sounding, the emergency never ends. Though people with PTSD strive to avoid any reminder of the traumatic event, they often find themselves reliving it. Around one in twenty people in England are currently living with PTSD. For women between sixteen and twenty-four the figure is almost 13 per cent.

Could traumatic events, I wondered, trigger paranoia? It

seemed highly probable. It was easy to imagine that trauma inflicted deliberately by other people (and often, of course, it isn't) could change the way we feel about ourselves and others, breeding anxiety about both our own vulnerability and the readiness of others to exploit that perceived weakness. As a first step towards answering that question, I included a trauma assessment among the battery of tests given to the two hundred participants in our virtual tube experiment. Seventy per cent of these Londoners described experiencing at least one traumatic event in their lifetime. A quarter reported having endured childhood physical or sexual abuse; 7.5 per cent had been victims of severe childhood sexual abuse. Working with the clinical psychologist David Fowler, a pioneer of CBT for psychosis and one of the first people to highlight the link with trauma, I found a very clear association between the experience of trauma and paranoid thinking. In fact, the likelihood of reporting persecutory ideas was two and a half times greater for people who had experienced trauma than for those fortunate enough to have been spared it. This was a cross-sectional study: a one-off snapshot relying on participants' memory of what in many cases had occurred several years before. So I couldn't be certain that trauma was causing paranoia. But the data did support the idea that, if there *were* a causal pathway from trauma to paranoia, that pathway might be anxiety. Horrible events can trigger long-lasting fear about what ill-intentioned people might want to inflict upon us.

Revealing though it was, my virtual tube study was dwarfed in scale by the 2007 Adult Psychiatric Morbidity Survey. The APMS interviewed more than seven thousand people, representative of the general population in England. As we saw in Chapter 4, my analysis of the APMS data had shown that paranoia was widespread. To the question 'Over the past year, have there been times when you felt that people were against you?', 18.6 per cent answered positively. Eight per cent stated that there had been times when they'd felt that people were deliberately acting to harm them. Almost 2 per cent said they'd thought a group of people were plotting to cause them serious harm or injury. When I looked at the trauma data in the APMS, the association with paranoia was unmistakeable. Indeed, the chance of people with a potential PTSD diagnosis reporting severe paranoia was *twenty-seven times* the likelihood for those without such a diagnosis.

Reactions to an assault

'*Every year several thousand people pass through the Accident and Emergency Department after an assault. This study concerns reactions to the assault over the next six months. We want to find out how many people have difficulties coping with the incident (e.g. remain distressed by it) and how many people are relatively unaffected by the incident (e.g. rarely think about it). Importantly, we want to identify the factors that may lead to the different reactions.*'
                                        Instructions to study participants

It's clear that trauma and paranoia are closely connected. But does the former cause the latter? Proving it is tricky. We can't experimentally allocate a traumatic event to some people and not others to see what happens. Nevertheless, the APMS survey and the tube study data certainly suggested a causal relationship: if you had experienced trauma, there was a good chance that you'd develop paranoia. But why? I suspected that the explanation might lie in the psychological reaction to trauma. In order to find out, though, a cross-sectional study wouldn't work. Instead, we needed to take a longitudinal approach, following people over a number of months to see how their thoughts and feelings evolved. So in 2010 I teamed up with Anke Ehlers, one of the world leaders in PTSD research and treatment. We recruited 106 adults who had been admitted in the previous four weeks to the A&E Department at King's College Hospital in London following an assault.

The stories told by the participants were sobering. Many had been attacked in some kind of confrontation. They had tried to break up a fight, for example, but ended up on the receiving end themselves. Almost a quarter had been the victims of a random attack. I remember one man who had been set upon from behind by a group of boys while walking down a busy street. Twenty-two had been violently mugged, like the woman who had been punched after refusing to surrender her bag. Nineteen had been involved in one-off arguments with a friend or family member, and eight had been attacked while at work. One unlucky support worker had been assaulted by the boy she'd been looking after. These attacks had resulted in some pretty serious injuries, with only four of the 106 escaping with just minor cuts and bruises. Seven had been beaten into unconsciousness. Four suffered damage to their internal organs. More than a quarter had broken bones. A third sustained a head injury. Seventy-one were left with major cuts and bruises.

Most of these incidents had happened near where I was then living. Hearing about them certainly dented my rather happy-go-lucky attitude to London life. I spent a lot more time checking behind me when I was out and about. And I avoided the park after dark. An over-reaction, or a rational response to risk? It's a question that was even more pertinent for our A&E study. After all, is it fair to use the term 'paranoid' in relation to someone who has been assaulted? If they've become fearful of other people isn't that entirely reasonable? Isn't it an adaptive strategy to prevent further harm? Well, it depends. What we wanted to capture was the *generalisation* of fear: the process by which a particular, possibly helpful anxiety broadens into a pervasive, debilitating dread. (In Cosslett's case, fear of another assault grew into a conviction that the entire world was trying to kill her.)

Distinguishing between justified fear and excessive mistrust is difficult at the best of times, but when you're working with people who've undergone trauma it can be especially challenging. So, with research assistants Claire Thompson and Natasha Vorontsova, we carried out what I suspect is the most comprehensive assessment of paranoia ever undertaken. We first met our participants four weeks after their admission to A&E. We assessed them for both PTSD and paranoia, and we did so again three and six months later. That paranoia evaluation included standard questionnaires, for which we reminded participants not to include thoughts or feelings about the person who had assaulted them. They also took a ride on our virtual London tube train. As you may remember from Chapter 4, we'd populated the tube carriage with computer-generated characters programmed to behave neutrally – no friendliness and no aggression, just deadpan indifference. If someone reported hostility from an avatar, we knew that what we were hearing was paranoia. But this wasn't all we did by way of assessment. We also spent a lot of time talking with our participants, trying to establish whether they believed their fears had got out of hand – whether, for example, they were now fearful of all males or frightened to be out of the house at any time. We used these interviews to rate the participant's paranoia, rather than simply relying on their own self-report. And we made sure that when we did so, we excluded fears about the perpetrators of their assault.

What did we learn? Four weeks after being assaulted, a third of the group displayed symptoms consistent with a diagnosis of PTSD. Six months later, that number had declined to 16 per cent. Those figures are what we'd expect after an attack. As for paranoia, rates were very high. For example, at four weeks, 80 per cent of the group reported that they were now excessively frightened of other people. Around 10 per cent appeared to have clinical levels of paranoia. We'd used various measures of paranoia: all of them told the same story. As the months passed, that elevated level of mistrust fell – but not by much. At the end of the study two-thirds of people were still prone to paranoid thoughts. It's possible, of course, that some of the participants had been exhibiting significant paranoia before they were assaulted. If not – and certainly many of the group participants believed that the incident had made them more suspicious – what we see here is the lasting effect of trauma on levels of trust. Our participants weren't simply worried about another assault. They became generally fearful of other people, especially men. Moreover, the way in which an individual responded psychologically to their assault didn't only predict whether they'd develop PTSD. It was also strongly linked to paranoia. So let's look now at the kind of reaction that can turn trauma into PTSD – and trust into paranoia.

'People can't be trusted'

Not everyone develops PTSD after an assault. And not everyone ends up with a generalised mistrust of other people. Why? What makes the difference?

As you might expect, the nature of the trauma is important. PTSD is more likely if the trauma is severe, long-lasting, unpredictable, and suffered at the hands of other people. When it comes to paranoia, our A&E study showed that some assaults were especially damaging – though not, as it happens, the ones we had expected. We had hypothesised that being attacked by a stranger while away from home would be most likely to breed general mistrust. Almost all people and places could then seem threatening. But in fact the opposite was true. Being attacked close to home, or by someone the individual knew, was more likely to trigger paranoia. This is perhaps because these kinds of incident most radically violate our expectations of safety. Most of us trust that, when we're with people we know, or when we're at home, we are secure. Being assaulted in such situations destroys that trust.

But it's not that simple. What matters isn't only the event, but how we make sense of it. The psychological impact of even the most distressing situations is determined, at least in part, by our reaction – by how we think, feel and behave, both during the traumatic event and afterwards. (This emphatically does not mean, however, that psychological problems are somehow our fault. There are almost always entirely understandable reasons for why we respond as we do in a given situation.)

Thanks to the pioneering work of Anke Ehlers and David Clark, we know what kinds of response are most likely to develop into PTSD. Ehlers and Clark argue that PTSD is rooted in a belief that, though the traumatic event is over, we are still in danger. Why does this happen? There are two main reasons. One is to do with memory; the other stems from the way we view ourselves and the world around us. Let's start with memory. PTSD springs from a memory of the event that is unrooted. It's like 'a cupboard in which many things have been thrown in quickly and in a disorganised fashion, so it is impossible to fully close the door and things fall out at unpredictable times'. In other words, because we haven't properly processed the memory, it's liable to intrude at any time. The slightest sensory reminder of the trauma – a colour, a smell, a vague physical resemblance – can be enough. When that happens, the distinction between past and present dissolves. We are transported back into the traumatic situation. Rhiannon Lucy Cosslett: 'Something flips and I am back there, on the pavement with his hands around my neck, screaming.' We can't make sense of what has happened. We can't control our memories of it. And therefore we can't move on with our life. For our A&E group, unwanted memories weren't just a feature of PTSD. They were also clearly linked to persistent paranoia.

How should we deal with distressing memories? People with PTSD try to bolt the cupboard door closed. They don't want to think about their suffering. They don't want to talk about it. Instead, they seek erasure. It's an understandable strategy when memories are so painful. But it doesn't work. Even worse, it actually makes those memories *more* likely to intrude. If you doubt it, for the next couple of minutes try thinking about whatever you like apart from a huge yellow elephant. Difficult, isn't it? That elephant keeps on coming to mind. So we can't make peace with painful memories by pretending they don't exist. Thought suppression merely ensures that those memories bounce right back. In the case of our A&E group, remembering their assault – over and over again – also reinforced their fear of other people.

Alongside memory, the other critical factor in the development of both PTSD and paranoia is the damage done by trauma to our view of ourselves and the people around us. Here are some of the statements endorsed on a self-report scale by many of our A&E group:

'I am inadequate.'
'I can't stop bad things from happening to me.'
'I have permanently changed for the worse.'
'People can't be trusted.'
'You never know who will harm you.'
'The world is a dangerous place.'

These are of course very categorical statements. The fear, and the self-reproach, has generalised into a simple binary proposition: I am weak and vulnerable; others are powerful and cruel. If we think like this, mistrust doesn't seem so unreasonable. In fact, it can feel like the only thing standing between us and more trauma. And it's easy to assume we need its protection round the clock. After all, if we never know who will harm us, we can never really let our guard down. We're always ready to take evasive action.

Some of the participants in our study may have had these pessimistic thoughts before they were assaulted. But such beliefs are often a consequence of how people feel *during* the traumatic event. Key here is a sense of personal defeat. 'I didn't feel like I was a human being any more . . . Mentally, I gave up . . . I'm a loser'. As Ehlers and Clark say: 'Patients who experienced mental defeat are more likely than other victims to interpret the trauma as evidence for a negative view of themselves, for example, that they are unable to cope with stress, that they are not a worthy person or that they are permanently damaged by the trauma.' It is easy to imagine that feeling utterly vanquished – physically, psychologically, emotionally – could grow into a sense of extreme personal vulnerability. If we're incapable of defending ourselves, what chance do we have of preventing something awful from reoccurring?

Trauma doesn't only alter our memories and the way we think about ourselves and others. It can determine how we behave too. Usually this means staying away from the places or people that trigger upsetting memories. But it can also spark a kind of hypervigilance, a constant monitoring of the environment for signs of danger. Our A&E participants, for example, told us: 'I make sure I can always see what is going on'; 'I make sure I have a telephone near me so that I can call for help'; 'I check whether the people around me look suspicious'; 'I make extra efforts to make sure my surroundings are safe'. Ploys like these are what I call defences, and they're extremely common in PTSD, in anxiety disorders – and in paranoia too. (Remember Robert in Chapter 1, hiding at the rear of the house lest he be observed by the government.)

The assault victims who developed paranoia may have sought to avoid any reminder of their ordeal. It may have been the very last thing they wanted to think about. And yet it gnawed away at them. Again and again, whether because of an involuntary memory or a conscious decision, their minds would come back to the incident that had brought them to King's College Hospital. This persistent rumination on what has happened in the past, and worry about what may occur in the future, is typical of PTSD. *How could this horrible situation have been avoided? What should I have done differently? How will I cope if I have to go through it all over again?* Worry and rumination transport us back to the moment of trauma, reigniting feelings of pain, fear and despair, and colouring our sense of both past and future. In the case of an assault, we return to a world defined by our own vulnerability and the brutality of others. Of course, these patterns of thinking don't just fuel PTSD. They are exactly the kind of thoughts to stoke paranoia too.

Toxic environments

'I had an Instagram page that I made of my favourite band and it allowed me to make friends online with similar interests, but when people from school found the page, I ended up getting so much grief. People saw I was different and expressing myself and didn't like it, because I didn't fit in, they would call me all sorts of names. I would just feel like an outcast and that people would hold that against me. I just didn't want

to be there, school just seemed like such a toxic environment. Walking past a group of boys, it takes me back to when I was in school, and I worry if they are going to say something.'

'I was bullied by my boss. She and my co-worker would whisper, go out together for lunch and not invite me, laugh at each other's jokes and stare dumbly when I would try to join in – all the petty ways to make you feel small and stupid. She would also hold private meetings with me where she would attack my character, my ability and my performance. Sometimes she would ask me to do something and then criticise me for doing it, trying to say she'd never asked me to do that task. I suffered extreme anxiety and would dread returning to work the moment I left.'

No matter how many years have passed, I'll bet that you can recall your school bullies. The kids you did your best to avoid. The ones who sought out the vulnerable and made their lives a misery. The ones who perhaps made *your* life a misery. Memories like that linger. Around a third of people have been bullied at school. For some, the experience never really leaves them. And bullying is not confined to school years. Globally, at least one in ten people are bullied in the workplace, and the figure may be as high as one in five.

Bullying enacts a crude and often brutal power relationship in which the victim is humiliated by an apparently invincible aggressor. Predictably, its effects on mental health can be devastating. Anxiety, depression, suicidal thoughts, PTSD: all have been persuasively linked to bullying. It turns out that it is also a significant factor in paranoia. In a study led by Gennaro Catone at the University of Naples, we analysed data from the 2000 and 2007 UK Adult Psychiatric Morbidity Surveys – all in all, sixteen thousand members of the general population. In both surveys those who'd been subjected to bullying, whether as a child or an adult, were more likely to experience the serious persecutory delusions that are so common in psychosis. As we've seen, snapshot surveys like the APMS are not normally designed to detect causation: what they do is capture associations. But the 2000 APMS included an eighteen-month follow-up for a proportion of the original sample. That follow-up data showed that the link between bullying and paranoia wasn't merely associational. The former predicted the latter. In fact, bullying doubled the risk of developing paranoia – which isn't surprising given the sense of vulnerability it can so easily instil. If this person can behave so cruelly towards me, we might easily wonder, what's to stop others from doing the same?

On the face of it, bullying is a perfect example of the way in which random malevolence can wreck our wellbeing, warping our sense of ourselves and others. But in fact, chance is less influential than we might assume, at least in some instances. Research led by Angelica ('Geli') Ronald at Birkbeck's Centre for Brain and Cognitive Development suggests that being bullied, and the paranoia to which it can lead, may be partly the result of genetics. Geli analysed data on almost five thousand twins from the Twins Early Development Study (TEDS) born in England and Wales between 1994 and 1996. Twin studies like Geli's are a powerful way to gauge genetic influence, thanks to the differences between fraternal (or 'dizygotic') and identical ('monozygotic') twins. Fraternal twins develop from separate eggs fertilised by separate sperm. Like all siblings, fraternal twins share 50 per cent of their genes. Identical (or 'monozygotic') twins, however, have exactly the same DNA: they are the result of a single egg, fertilised by a single sperm, dividing in two. If rates of a psychological disorder are more similar in identical twins than fraternal twins, we can be reasonably sure that this is down to their genes.

Looking at the TEDS data, Geli found a modest link between childhood bullying and subsequent paranoia: if you'd experienced the former you were more likely to develop the latter. No surprise there. More remarkable, however, was the contribution of genes both to the likelihood of being bullied and to subsequent paranoia. For bullying, heritability was 35 per cent; in the case of paranoia, it stood at 52 per cent. Most interesting of all, though, the link between being bullied and later paranoia was almost entirely explained by shared genetic influences. In other words, there is a genetic predisposition that raises the risk both of being bullied and of having paranoid thoughts.

What does that heritability figure signify? What it *doesn't* mean is that 35 per cent of a person's susceptibility to bullying is a result of their genes. Instead it tells us that 35 per cent of the *differences* in levels of susceptibility *across the population* are probably genetic in origin. Imagine a country in which the adult population ranges between five and six feet tall – and where heritability for height is 10 per cent. This isn't an improbable land in which genes play virtually no part in determining how tall people are. But it does seem that people *vary* in height largely because of environmental causes. And there's something else we must bear in mind when it comes to heritability. In this hypothetical country, the prime minister is five foot eleven while their partner is five foot exactly. What percentage of that eleven-inch difference between the two can we attribute to genetic factors? We've no way of knowing. It could be all or nothing or any point in between. The heritability figure tells us nothing about individuals. What it captures is population-wide patterns.

This was just one study, to be sure, but it does seem that certain children are more likely to be bullied than others – and to go on to develop paranoia. And part of the reason for this is genetic. It's what's known as a gene–environment correlation, in which our life experiences are influenced by genetic factors.

So what genetic factors are at play in bullying? One may well be personality. For most of us, personality is pretty stable. It doesn't tend to change a great deal, at least by the time we're adults. So, how much of that stability is due to our genes? Some scientists have argued that personality is essentially a product of biological factors determined by our DNA. Hans Eysenck, for instance, believed that a person's level of extraversion was a function of their nervous system. Indeed, there's some evidence that very extrovert people possess relatively insensitive physiologies. That means they tend to seek out strong sensory stimulation, whether that's partying, playing competitive sports, or climbing mountains (research suggests both professional athletes and climbers are high in extroversion). People who score highly for introversion, on the other hand, require much less stimulation and hence are content with less adventurous pursuits. Not everyone buys this strongly biological account of personality. But the current best guess is that heritability for personality is around 40 to 50 per cent. So there's clearly a significant genetic element. And when it comes to bullying, children who are perceived to be introverted, anxious and unsure of themselves may be especially at risk. As it happens, these are also traits that are common in people prone to paranoia.

Personality isn't of course the only way in which genes can increase vulnerability to bullying. In 2016 UNICEF surveyed 100,000 young people in eighteen countries around the world. Two-thirds reported that they'd been the victim of bullying. A quarter of those young people said that they had been singled out because of their physical appearance (other studies have found this to be the number one factor). A quarter attributed the bullying to their ethnicity or nationality. (Immigrant children, for example, are especially vulnerable.) And another 25 per cent felt that their gender or sexual orientation made them targets. LGBT children often endure particularly high levels of harassment: a study in New Zealand, for instance, found that lesbian, gay or bisexual students were three times as likely to be bullied as heterosexual young people, and transgender students five times. In all these cases, what we see in bullying is the punishment of perceived difference. And this fits with other evidence indicating that people who have suffered discrimination are more likely to report paranoid thoughts. Although the precise genetic influence on, say, physical appearance or ethnicity or sexuality will vary, there's no doubt that it's generally a significant influence.

More evidence for the link between bullying and paranoia arose from a study led by the clinical psychologist (and my PhD student at the time) Jessica Bird. In 2019 Jess returned to her old secondary school in Leicestershire and gathered data from eight hundred students aged eleven to fifteen. Sadly, paranoia looked to be pretty widespread. For example, 32 per cent of students regularly worried about what strangers might do to them. Thirty per cent thought, at least twice a week, that other people were deliberately lying to them. A quarter frequently suspected that people at school were trying to make them feel unwanted. Twenty-three per cent believed they might be attacked at any time, and one in five said they felt unsafe wherever they went. As far as we know, there was nothing extraordinary about this group. The Leicestershire secondary could have been, presumably, more or less any school in the UK. The young people could have been any young people.

The teenagers who reported these paranoid thoughts were more likely to say that they had been bullied. But victimisation was just one of a number of unhappy experiences clustered around paranoia. These young people slept badly. They worried about their body image. They struggled to build firm friendships. Fundamentally, they were at least somewhat depressed and anxious. It was these emotional problems that likely left the young people vulnerable to other difficulties, including paranoia. We've seen this a lot in adults too: low mood primes mistrust. (We'll dive into the detail of this in Chapter 8.) As self-confidence wavers, fear grows. The world begins to seem a dismal, dangerous place. Resilience, on the other hand, feels paper-thin.

Among adults, overall rates of paranoia are similar for men and women. That said, there are significant differences. Men are more likely than women to endorse relatively severe suspicious thoughts (for example, 'In the past year, have there been times when you felt that a group of people was plotting to cause you serious harm or injury?'). Women, on the other hand, show higher rates of relatively mild paranoia ('Over the past year, have there been times when you felt that people were against you?'). Among the Leicestershire teenagers, however, paranoia was especially acute for the girls. This was not a surprise. Girls tend to be more socially anxious than boys, more worried about social exclusion, and less trusting. And there is perhaps no time in our lives when social relationships matter more, and yet seem so difficult to navigate, than adolescence. More generally, rates of anxiety and depression are much higher – some studies suggest twice as high – in adolescent females than males.

Then there is the matter of the harassment and violence to which women are routinely subjected. By way of a few examples from a sorry mass of data on the topic: in 2021 the UK All-Party Parliamentary Group (APPG) for UN Women reported that 71 per cent of women in the UK have experienced some form of sexual harassment in a public space. Among 18 to 24-year-olds, that number was 86 per cent. Only 3 per cent of this younger age group said they'd never been harassed in any way. In the US, more than one in five women reported having suffered completed or attempted rape at some point in their lifetime. Eighty per cent of those cases happened before the age of twenty-five. Forty-three per cent of women had experienced sexual violence, defined as rape, sexual coercion or unwanted sexual contact. Given these statistics, it's not difficult to see why the most common paranoid fear among the Leicestershire teenagers focused on what strangers might do to them.

'They're going to kill me'

What endemic sexual harassment and violence can do to young women's view of the world was amply demonstrated by Jess's conversations with twelve adolescents, aged eleven to seventeen, attending mental health services in our local NHS trust. The twelve – three boys and nine girls – were chosen because of their high levels of paranoia and drawn from a group of three hundred we had assessed in a larger study.

Those three hundred young people had largely been attending services for anxiety and depression. But they also showed high rates of paranoia. More than half thought that people were deliberately lying to them. Over 40 per cent were fearful of strangers. And 35 per cent felt unsafe everywhere around people. Overall, rates were twice as high as in the Leicestershire school group. Yet paranoia did not feature as a problem in their clinical notes and only one young person had discussed their fears with a therapist. It was another reminder that, even among mental health professionals, we still haven't really grasped just how common excessive mistrust is, nor how it meshes with other psychological problems.

Again, paranoia was much more common among the girls in Oxfordshire than the boys. Forty-one per cent reported at least mildly elevated levels; for boys, the figure was 'just' 24 per cent. Once more fears about personal safety loomed large. In fact, every single one of the twelve young people we interviewed worried that other people, primarily strangers, would physically harm them. Ten of the group were afraid that they might be kidnapped. Five of the nine girls feared sexual assault by men:

> When you always hear things on the news and there's so much of it going on nowadays, and your mother's always warning you and your grandparents are always warning you, it's just so difficult to not have those thoughts. Especially as I'm female, I'm not being sexist, but they're more targeted for assault and stuff. (Chloe, 14)

> I don't trust men . . . When they're too close to you, I'm like 'oh my god, they're going to take me, they're going to kidnap me, someone's setting on me, they're going to kill me.' (Katie, 16)

It's worth bearing in mind here that, though women are routinely subject to sexual violence, when it comes to physical attacks, young males are also – and perhaps especially – at risk. Hence perhaps the worrying, albeit lower, level of paranoia among the boys. The UK Office for National Statistics, for example, reported in March 2022 that men were more likely to be the victims of violent crime than women (2.2 per cent of men compared to 1.6 per cent of women) – though they also note that domestic violence is significantly under-reported. Younger people tend to be at greater risk than older people. In the ONS survey 3 per cent of 18 to 24-year-olds and 2.9 per cent of 25 to 34-year-olds reported experiencing violent crimes, compared to 0.6 per cent of those aged 65 to 74, for example.

As we grow up, we discover that the world is not always as benign as it may have seemed when we were younger. According to sixteen-year-old Sophie: 'You're kind of like, I've got the world to grow into, but it's not something safe. It's something

I've got to always be careful of because I'm not going to be able to protect myself . . . It's a lot more scary because you know you're growing up and you're going to be facing things more independently, [but] you don't really know how to deal with it.' Like Chloe, one of the lessons we learn from our family, our friends, and the media is that men can be volatile, unpleasant and physically dangerous, and that women are particularly vulnerable. Megan, also sixteen, said, 'Sometimes it makes me feel dirty, because all the men come up to me, and I feel like I look like a slag and stuff.' And girls in particular come to understand that they must amend their behaviour accordingly: where they go, who they go with, and how they behave while they're there (even down to the clothes they wear). Stay vigilant. Suspect others. *Be careful.*

The young people Jess Bird spoke to in Oxfordshire were only too aware of the damage done by excessive fear:

I should be able to go out with my friends and enjoy my time, I shouldn't have to worry about being kidnapped or murdered or anything else, because I'm only fifteen, I'm still very young and I shouldn't have to grow up with these worries. I should be able to enjoy my life while I can. (Holly, 15)

It's not really that nice because I can see people on social media going out to their friends' parties and things like that, or just spending time together and I just don't have trust in people to do that . . . I get really sad at home, and I'm like, oh, I want to get out, but when I do I just get really panicky so I just don't bother. (Emily, 16)

The challenge, and for sure it's a difficult one, is to help young people develop the skills they require to remain safe while simultaneously empowering them to lead the lives they choose.

Even more importantly, can we curb the behaviour of males that puts so many adolescents – and adults – at risk?

I will leave the last word in this chapter to Rhiannon Lucy Cosslett. After months of cognitive behaviour therapy, and with medication, Cosslett's paranoia and PTSD passed:

I go outside again. I take a plane. I sit in a square in the sun. I go to bars and out to eat. I get the tube in rush hour. I no longer live with the contradiction of fearing death while at the same time wanting to throw myself in front of oncoming traffic in order to stop that ever-present fear. It feels like a miracle.

6.

In the blood?

'All of them. Or at least practically all of them. Especially the teenagers. They don't like me, so they try to wind me up.'

Michael Allen was sixty years old, married with several grown-up children, and working part time in an insurance company. We met at my weekly NHS clinic in Croydon, south London (when I was still at the Institute of Psychiatry). As we talked, his eyes darted nervously around the consulting room, as if he were expecting trouble at any moment or looking for an escape route.

'How do they try to wind you up?'

'They shout at me. They laugh at me. Sometimes they bump into me on the street.'

'Can you think of a recent example?'

'It happened this morning. On the bus coming to see you.'

'What happened?'

'I was sitting downstairs at the front of the bus. I don't like going upstairs on my own and I don't like to sit at the back. I could hear these kids getting at me. I don't know what they found so funny, but they were giggling and laughing and heaven knows what else. I should be used to it by now, I suppose, but it really upset me.'

'What made you think they were laughing at you? Is it at all possible that there was another explanation?'

'I suppose so.' He gave a sheepish but determined smile. 'But I know. I just know.'

'Why do you think young people pick on you?'

He paused and, once again, looked around the room.

'I don't know. Maybe I'm a soft target. Or maybe someone's put a curse on me. I was a difficult child. A bit stroppy. Not very nice sometimes. Perhaps I'm being punished for that.'

By the time I met him, Mr Allen had been experiencing paranoid thoughts for thirty years. These days his mistrust tended to be focused on local young people. But he also believed that his neighbours had installed surveillance equipment in his house in order to annoy him. His wife and family were sure he was mistaken. They'd seen no evidence to support his interpretation of events. And yet Mr Allen was absolutely convinced that he was being persecuted. In our first meeting I asked him to rate, on a scale of 0 to 100, how strongly he believed his thoughts. Without hesitation, and with a vigorous nod of the head, he answered: 'One hundred per cent.'

Mr Allen lived his fears day and night. They were a perpetual presence, a constant preoccupation. 'They just pop into my head. I could be watching TV, or cooking, or getting ready for bed and suddenly there they are. I can't control them. They control me.'

'I'm guessing these thoughts make you feel bad?'

'Awful. Sick to the stomach. Sad. Like I want to cry.'

Because he only felt safe at home, Mr Allen had become increasingly reluctant to leave the house without his wife. 'I feel like a prisoner,' he told me. 'But what else can I do?' Going to work had become a real challenge; some days he just couldn't face it. So now, to add to his worries, Mr Allen dreaded losing his job. 'And then what'll happen to me? At my age and with my history, I'll never work again.' He rarely saw people socially: 'If you don't get out much, pretty soon you're forgotten. Friends move on, don't they? I don't blame them. No one wants to deal with this stuff.' Worst of all, he was wracked by guilt at the 'burden' his wife had carried for so many years. 'It's so hard for her. She deserves better. She deserves a normal life. It breaks my heart.'

The isolation Mr Allen was describing is common among people with psychosis. Many of the patients I see are single. Many have – at best – only a small social network to look to for support (usually comprising family members). This is often true even for people experiencing their first psychotic episode. For example, in a study led by Oliver Sündermann, one-third of people being treated for a first episode of psychosis in south London said they had no one with whom to share their thoughts and feelings. Again, this isn't unusual. Other research has suggested that people newly diagnosed with psychosis are seven times more likely to lack a confidant than the rest of the population. On average, Sündermann's group – mostly young and male – saw friends or family only four times per week. Not everyone needs lots of social contact, of course, and quality is more important than quantity. But the people in Sündermann's study regularly felt lonely, and the lonelier they felt the more psychiatric problems they experienced.

In his concern for his wife, Mr Allen highlighted another typical consequence of psychosis: the toll taken on carers. We can hear their voices in much-needed work led by Andrés Estradé and Juliana Onwumere, and in a separate Australian project by Terence McCann and colleagues. In most cases the role of carer is assumed by close relatives, often parents or partners. No one is prepared for the upheaval diagnosis brings: 'Nothing in her growing-up years could have prepared us for the shock and devastation of seeing this normal, happy child become totally incapacitated by schizophrenia. . . . What we knew about schizophrenia, in the beginning, we could have written on the head of a pin.' In the desperate attempt to make sense of what is happening to their loved one, carers can become wracked by guilt: 'I blamed myself. It had to be someone's fault.' It can feel as if you're living with a stranger: 'The woman who was once attractive, confident, kind, discerning, and popular became a social recluse, a sullen figure, and a "mumbler" of paranoid notions.' The sense of loss can be acute: 'Although grieving for someone who has died is painful, some sense of peace and acceptance is ultimately possible. However, mourning for a loved one who is alive – in your very presence and yet in vital ways inaccessible to you – has a lonely, unreal quality that is extraordinarily painful.' Where did that person go? When, if ever, will they return? 'I treasure the times Cindy looks at me and tells me I'm beautiful when she tells me my dress is pretty [. . .]. This is the "real" Cindy speaking – my sweet, generous, funny, intelligent daughter.'

Like the person with psychosis, carers can find that their world shrinks dramatically: 'Our social life was the first thing that changed noticeably. When we were with friends or relatives, my husband started making embarrassing remarks when he thought he heard them conspiring against him [. . .] Gradually, most of our friends drifted away.' It can be easy to feel that you're on your own: 'In this new situation of a mental health problem, I had neither love nor support, and did not know where to find help. There was no one with whom I could share this burden. The whole territory of mental health problems was strange, unpredictable and frightening.' And it is exhausting: 'it's very physically, emotionally and mentally straining. The stress that it causes me is just too much.'

Things are often made even tougher by the perception that people with psychosis don't receive the help they need from health services: '[I'm] just frustrated and worn out with it all. Just, I can't say I blame an individual; I think it's the system as a whole. [. . .] I really don't think you should have to hit rock bottom before somebody does something.' When 'something' is eventually done, carers can feel frozen out – 'I felt that I was invisible, as nobody seemed to notice me' – when what they want to be is listened to and guided by professionals to assist in their loved one's treatment: 'I am convinced that if someone had helped me understand my husband's illness without my having to go through the long, painful process of learning step by step, and if I had been made aware of my own weaknesses before being drawn into inescapable vicious circles, much pain could have been avoided.'

Virtually every day I am contacted by carers asking how they can get help – both for themselves and their loved one. Or wanting to know where to turn when a family member is refusing treatment. Sometimes the situation is even more fraught because in the person's paranoia the carer isn't an ally but a threat. What do you do when your loved one seems to have turned against you? When they suspect that you are spying on them, or maligning them to others, or secretly adding medication to their food? Nevertheless, there is no doubt that the love and support of carers can make all the difference to patients: 'My immediate family is the greatest asset I have and the most important aspect of my life. They know who I am and accept me every bit. They have supported me throughout the illness, and they are supporting me as I get back on my feet to lead a "normal life".'

Is mistrust genetic?

Mr Allen had endured a difficult childhood. His parents, he recalled, had struggled to bring up six children with very little money. 'They had it tough. Always working several jobs, both

of them. But it was fine – you know, the kids kind of looked
after each other. And we didn't know any different. No one was
to blame – it was just one of those things. I've no complaints.'
But things were perhaps not as fine as all that. What all the
children lacked, Mr Allen said, was attention from their parents.
'We didn't see a lot of them, because they were usually out
working. And when they were home, they were exhausted. So
not much conversation and all that.' Mr Allen must, I imagine,
have sometimes felt overlooked, a cast-off in a world that seemed
largely indifferent to his fate. Did this early adversity prepare
the ground for his later paranoia? Should we look even further
back to vulnerabilities inherited via his genes? What part, if
any, do genetics play in mistrust? Is paranoia simply a product
of our life experiences?

There is a centuries-old view that severe mental health disorders are primarily biological in origin: that they are the
consequence of brain defects, damage or disease. It's an argument that has often dominated thinking about mental health,
and it remains highly influential today. Long before the discovery
of DNA, there were those who argued that 'cerebral infirmities'
could be transmitted from parent to child. In the late nineteenth
century, this thinking had a distinctly eugenicist spin:

> The insane neurosis which the child inherits in consequence
> of its parent's insanity is as surely a defect of physical nature
> as is the epileptic neurosis to which it is so closely allied.
> It is an indisputable though extreme fact that certain human
> beings are born with such a native deficiency of mind that
> all the training and education in the world will not raise
> them to the height of brutes; and I believe it to be not less
> true that, in consequence of evil ancestral influences, indi-
> viduals are born with such a flaw or warp of nature that
> all the care in the world will not prevent them from being

vicious or criminal, or becoming insane. . . . No one can escape the tyranny of his organization; no one can elude the destiny that is innate in him . . .

This was the leading British psychiatrist Henry Maudsley writing in 1873. (Maudsley had 'induced the London County Council by a contribution of thirty thousand pounds to build a hospital for the early treatment of mental disease'. That hospital, where I worked for so long, was finally opened in 1923 – sixteen years after Maudsley had first approached the LCC and five years after his death.) Maudsley was an energetic advocate of mental health care, publishing numerous influential books, lobbying successfully for the inclusion in medical degrees of a mandatory course in mental health, and introducing a national training scheme for psychiatric nurses. But his determination to increase access to treatment coexisted with a bleakly determinist perspective on the causes of mental health problems. He was not alone in this kind of thinking: the idea was rife in Victorian society. Like some biblical prophet, Thomas Arnold, headmaster of Rugby School, decreed: 'It is the law of God's providence which we cannot alter, that the sins of the father are really visited upon the child in the corruption of his breed.' In Maudsley's view, those individuals who inherited a predisposition to psychiatric conditions could be cared for by physicians. They could lessen the chances of their children suffering the same fate by a judicious choice of mate. But were the 'morbid predisposition' to continue through the family, Nature would eventually intervene. Descendants would become infertile, thereby averting the 'permanent degradation of the race'.

That serious psychological problems were often biological in origin was a fundamental tenet of the fledgling science of psychiatry, which as we saw in Chapter 3 structured itself around a distinction between neuroses (anxiety and depression, for instance) and psychoses. Neuroses, you may remember, were seen as psychological problems caused by life experiences. Psychoses were understood as the result of biological disease. Writing in 1913, Karl Jaspers cautioned psychiatrists against mistaking one for the other:

> Pathological symptoms are layered like an onion, with degenerative symptoms . . . forming the outmost layer, moving inwards to the process symptoms (schizophrenias) and finally the innermost layers comprising organically based symptoms. The deepest layer reached in the course of examining an individual case is decisive. What initially appears to be a case of hysteria turns out to be multiple sclerosis, suspected neurasthenia is actually paralysis, melancholic depression a [biological] process.

As we know, paranoia was regarded as a psychotic symptom and thus the result of physical disease.

The enthusiasm for biological explanations of psychological phenomena never really went away. But it was hugely boosted by the advent of modern genetic science (and by the development in the 1970s of brain scanners). Mapping of the human genome was completed in 2003. Hundreds of genes involved in physical disease have been identified. But progress has been much slower for psychological disorders. No one now really believes that there are a few distinct genes causing, for example, depression or anxiety – the picture is far more complex. But it's clear that genes play a part in mental disorders, just as they do in most psychological characteristics. In the case of depression, for instance, heritability has been estimated at around 40 per cent. The figure is similar for anxiety disorders. For eating disorders, heritability is approximately 50 per cent. For alcohol disorders, it may be as high as 60 per cent. Remember though that this doesn't mean 40 per cent of a person's depression is necessarily genetic in origin. Rather it suggests that 40 per cent of the *differences* in levels of depression across, say, the UK are probably genetic. Heritability tells us nothing about individuals. What it reveals is population-wide patterns.

Some years back I found myself sitting next to the eminent behavioural geneticist Robert Plomin in a university committee meeting. During a pause in the proceedings, I told him I was interested to know whether genes contributed to paranoia. Many genetic studies of schizophrenia had been undertaken over the years, but I wanted to know about paranoia specifically. To what degree, I wondered, are people 'naturally' mistrustful? This was my rather transparent attempt at subtly testing the waters for a research collaboration. Luckily, Robert is naturally curious. 'Let's find out,' he said, and helpfully put me in touch with Geli Ronald, one of his former PhD students and then a rising star at Birkbeck's Centre for Brain and Cognitive Development.

With Geli most definitely at the helm, we analysed psychotic experiences in 5,059 adolescent pairs of twins from England and Wales taking part in Robert's Twins Early Development Study. What we found was a heritability figure for paranoia of 50 per cent. That is significantly lower than for a schizophrenia diagnosis, for which heritability is around 80 per cent. But it is similar to what we see in anxiety disorders. (Given the similarities between paranoia and anxiety, that may not be coincidental.) Strikingly, the TEDS study found that the severity of paranoia had no bearing on heritability. The same genes that help cause clinical-grade persecutory delusions are also likely to be at work in everyday mistrust. It's more support for the idea that paranoia, like other mental health problems, exists on a continuum. The paranoia experienced by people diagnosed with schizophrenia is simply an extreme example of everyday mistrust. The causes, and the factors that keep them going, are essentially alike.

We don't yet know which genes contribute to paranoia, though Geli has identified some potential candidates. Like other psychological disorders, however, when the picture eventually clarifies we're likely to find that many genes are involved. Individually, their influence may be small. Combined in a polygenic inheritance, however, the total of their contributions can be decisive. But if 50 per cent of the differences in levels of paranoia are due to genes, what about the other 50 per cent? The simplistic answer is that they are the result of environmental factors. Environment in this context is an extremely broad term, encompassing anything and everything that befalls us from the moment of conception. For paranoia, however, certain types of experience seem to be especially consequential. In a study led by Mark Taylor at Stockholm's Karolinska Institute, we went back to the TEDS data to look at the influence of five in particular: bullying; cannabis use; tobacco use; certain adverse life events such as a relationship breakdown or being the victim of a crime; and low birth weight. If you've read the previous chapter, you won't be surprised to hear about the impact of bullying or violent crime. But it turns out that all five of these life experiences were actually *more* important than genes in causing paranoia. (We'll discuss cannabis and tobacco in a later chapter, but in the case of low birth weight it seems the link with paranoia may lie in obstetric complications. These don't just sometimes lead to smaller babies, but may affect brain development too.) The same story emerged when we scrutinised data on 6,435 twin pairs from the Child and Adolescent Twin Study in Sweden. Some of us have a genetic susceptibility to paranoia. But without the life experiences that trigger suspicious thoughts that predisposition may remain latent (this is termed a gene–environment interaction). For others, damaging life experiences may be enough. If you've been bullied throughout your childhood, for example, there's a good chance that you'll be prone to paranoia. Your genetic make-up will be relatively unimportant.

Let's see what's under this box

'When a baby is born he cannot tell one person from another and indeed can hardly tell person from thing. Yet, by his first birthday he is likely to have become a connoisseur of people. Not only does he come quickly to distinguish familiars from strangers but amongst his familiars he chooses one or more favorites. They are greeted with delight; they are followed when they depart; and they are sought when absent. Their loss causes anxiety and distress; their recovery, relief and a sense of security. On this foundation, it seems, the rest of his emotional life is built . . .'
John Bowlby, psychiatrist and psychologist

We know that children learn fear from their parents. Indeed, they use adults' reactions as a guide to how they should respond in any given situation. This was neatly demonstrated in an experiment by Friederike Gerull and Ronald Rapee, who brought together thirty Australian toddlers, a green rubber snake – 90 centimetres long with its mouth open to reveal its fangs – and a black, green and purple rubber spider. The children's mothers were asked to reveal the toys – 'let's see what's under this box' – and to show either fear and disgust or happiness. Later the snake and spider were shown to the toddlers again, with their mothers remaining neutral in their reactions. It was easy to predict how the toddlers would respond. They reacted in the same way their mother had done first time around. If their mother had been upbeat and encouraging, so too was the child.

On the other hand, if their mother had shown fear or disgust, the toddler would avoid the toys.

Given how adeptly children assimilate the behaviour their parents model, it seems highly plausible that mistrust – which, after all, we can think of as a form of anxiety or fear – can also be learned. Those lessons may be delivered intentionally: through what is said, for instance. Or they can be inadvertently imparted through observation. But whether implicit or explicit, if we are taught as children that other people are unreliable, devious and dangerous, that world view may prove difficult to shake off. And the signs are that a great many of us may be growing up with this kind of perspective.

In 1997 a Danish woman was arrested in Manhattan. Her offence? Leaving her fourteen-month-old child to nap in a stroller outside the restaurant where she and her partner had stopped in for a drink. Anette Sørensen said she repeatedly checked on her daughter, who she could see through the restaurant window. But the police were called and both parents were charged with child endangerment. Sørensen was strip-searched and spent thirty-six hours in prison. In Denmark, Sørensen was perceived as a victim; in the US as a recklessly negligent mother. 'I had lived in New York [during school], so, of course, I knew that I didn't see prams all over the city,' Sørensen told the media. 'But . . . I had been living in Copenhagen, I had given birth to my daughter in Copenhagen, I was raised myself in Denmark . . . That's just how you do it in Denmark. People live in fear [in the US]. Children are not allowed to play in the playground alone.'

She may have a point. In 2021 researchers in the UK found that children were typically forbidden from playing outside unsupervised until the age of eleven. Their parents, on the other hand, reported that they had been allowed to do so by the age of nine. 'We can clearly see that there is a trend to be protective and to provide less freedom for our children now than in previous generations,' said Helen Dodd, the professor of child psychology at the University of Reading who led the study. Does it matter if kids don't get outside as much as older generations did? According to the NHS Health Survey for England, 10.1 per cent of reception age children (age 4–5) were obese in 2021/22. An additional 12.1 per cent were overweight. At age 10–11, 23.4 per cent were obese and 14.3 per cent overweight. And the trend is upwards. Obviously there are many factors in play here, but an increasingly sedentary lifestyle is likely to be one of them.

Moreover, playing outside isn't only critical for physical health. As Helen Dodd remarked: 'we are seeing children getting towards the end of their primary school years without having had enough opportunities to develop their ability to assess and manage risk independently.' It's conceivable that, in some cases, this will result in young people putting themselves in harm's way. Far more likely in my view is that they will grow up with an exaggerated sense of danger, to which mistrust becomes a reflex response. Indeed, in the UK fewer than half of people (46 per cent) in 2022 thought that most people can be trusted; for the US, the figure was just short of 40 per cent. These figures – and this fear – are highly contextual. In Sweden, for instance, almost two-thirds of respondents felt that most people could be trusted and in Norway it was almost three-quarters. (Ranking lowest in the latest iteration of the World Trust Survey was Zimbabwe, where just 2 per cent felt they could trust most people.)

Or take the perception of crime rates. In 2016 (the most recent year for which data are available), 60 per cent of UK adults thought that crime had increased over the previous twelve months. In fact, it had decreased by 6 per cent. In the US, Gallup's annual survey has shown that virtually every year most Americans believe that crime is rising despite it trending downwards. In 2022, 78 per cent of respondents thought that crime had gone up nationally. (It's possible that the US crime figures have indeed risen: they have yet to be issued. But given that perceptions of crime have little to do with the reality, this is probably neither here nor there.) Not only do we tend to overestimate the national crime rate, but we also have an exaggerated sense of our personal vulnerability. For example, 9 per cent of UK adults say that they are very worried about being robbed – thirty times higher than the actual crime rate (0.3 per cent of adults were victims of robbery in the year ending March 2016). Fifty-six per cent of Americans believed in 2022 that there was more crime in their locality than twelve months previously – the highest figure since 1972. Forty per cent worried about being mugged (up 7 per cent from the previous year); 36 per cent feared being attacked while driving (again, up 7 per cent); and 29 per cent were anxious about being murdered (up from 22 per cent).

It is plausible that adults with this pessimistic view of other people will tend to parent accordingly. Rather like the mothers in Gerull and Rapee's experiment, they may unconsciously model their anxiety. But they may also pursue a parenting style that other people would consider overprotective. Does heightened parental vigilance produce paranoid children? Poppy Brown, an outstanding doctoral student in my team at Oxford, set out to answer this question by analysing the results of the 2010 National Comorbidity Survey – Adolescents, a mammoth assessment of the mental health of over ten thousand US teenagers. Included in the NCS-A's battery of questions – so extensive that interviews took on average a gruelling two and a half hours – was a very brief measure of paranoia. Participants were asked whether they agreed with the statement: 'People often make fun of me behind my back'. (One question doesn't seem like much, and more would be better, but in fact this particular one is a reasonably effective means of gauging levels of paranoia.) Poppy then verified the results by conducting a survey of 1,286 adults in Oxfordshire.

Twenty-three per cent of the US participants, and 18 per cent of those in the UK, reported having paranoid ideas. It's yet another reminder of just how common this kind of thinking is among the general population. Sure enough, and especially in the US survey, this group was more likely to report that their parents had been excessively protective. Causation or correlation? For these data there's no way of knowing. This kind of research is very much a first step. But it seems credible that overprotective parenting could instil a sense of vulnerability in a child. If I weren't so helpless, and the world so dangerous, my mum and dad wouldn't need to worry about me so much, would they?

But other kinds of parenting may be even more influential when it comes to paranoia. They are unlikely to be sufficient on their own because psychological problems are almost always the product of multiple factors. And of course, many people who experience excessive mistrust will have had unproblematic upbringings. Nevertheless, in both the UK and US surveys, people who – like Mr Allen – reported that they had endured cold, uncaring or abusive parenting were much more likely to report having paranoid ideas. Most harmful of all in terms of trust were maternal indifference and paternal abuse (verbal or physical). For example, the odds of reporting paranoia were over four times higher for those who recalled experiencing a lot of paternal verbal abuse – defined as 'insulted or swore, shouted, yelled or screamed, threatened to hit' – compared to those who reported none. Again, Poppy Brown's study couldn't prove that these kinds of parenting produce paranoia in children. It offered a snapshot rather than a movie and snapshots aren't a good way of gauging the relationships between elements in a picture. But it seems likely. It is difficult to think of an experience that is as damaging to a child's self-esteem, or that sends such a clear message about other people's indifference and hostility.

It is worth bearing in mind, by the way, that this kind of parental behaviour appears to be more common than one might imagine. (Appears, because all we have to go on is what the survey participants reported. We can't corroborate their accounts.) Twenty-nine per cent of the US survey participants, and almost 18 per cent of the UK group, reported a lot of overprotective parenting by their mother. Occasional or frequent verbal abuse from a father figure, for example, was reported by 15 per cent of US adolescents and fully 25 per cent of the Oxfordshire group. Almost 16 per cent of the UK group (though just 4 per cent of US teenagers) said their father figure had sometimes or often 'pushed, grabbed or shoved, threw something, slapped or hit'.

When it comes to conspiracy theories, there is further evidence from a large US survey that upbringing matters. Working with Richard Bentall, a leading paranoia researcher at the University of Sheffield, I analysed data from 5,645 Americans interviewed in 2001–02 as part of the National Comorbidity Survey – Replication (NCS-R). A little over a quarter of the participants agreed with the statement: 'I am convinced there is a conspiracy behind many things in the world'. (This was, of course, long before the days of President Trump and QAnon.) These individuals were more likely to report having had potentially disruptive parental experiences during childhood, such as not living with both biological parents, or living away from home for an extended time. And they were more likely to describe having been frequently hit, pushed, grabbed, shoved, or having had something thrown at them in the home. Again, these experiences teach children that adults cannot be trusted; that they will put their own desires above the welfare of their children; and that they may even hurt them. The lesson is a grim one: I am vulnerable and even those closest to me may not hesitate to take advantage of that vulnerability. Is it any wonder then if mistrust results?

7.

'When I'm tired everything is worse'

'. . . at three o'clock in the morning a forgotten package has the same tragic importance as a death sentence, and the cure doesn't work . . . and in a real dark night of the soul it is always three o'clock in the morning, day after day.'
F. Scott Fitzgerald, *The Crack-Up* (1945)

'How has your sleep been? Do you sleep well most nights?'

Andrew puffs out his cheeks.

'Not great to be honest. Not too good at all.'

This isn't a surprise. Andrew looks exhausted. We're here to discuss his fears of harm at the hands of others, but from the dark circles under his eyes it's obvious that there are other problems we need to tackle too.

'How many hours sleep do you usually manage?'

He gives a wry smile.

'Not enough. It normally takes me ages to drop off. And then I'm awake a lot in the night. My mind is buzzing, worrying about this and that.'

'Do you sleep in the daytime?'

'Yeah,' Andrew nods. 'I don't want to – it screws up my day, you know, I can't get anything done. But I'm just so shattered.'

'Would you like us to work on improving your sleep?'

He answers immediately and decisively: 'Definitely. I'd really, really like that.' Andrew grins. 'When can we start?'

Most of the people I see in clinic are just like Andrew. They've been referred to me because of their paranoia, but they also aren't getting enough good-quality sleep. As we all know, that takes a toll. Just a few nights of broken sleep will likely make your mood plummet. You'll probably feel anxious and stressed and low. Everyday chores may morph into an impossible challenge. But though patients are well aware of the damage poor sleep does to their wellbeing – it's why our Feeling Safe treatment includes a module on improving sleep – most mental health professionals have been curiously slow to take on board this apparently self-evident truth. It's an oversight with deep roots.

Breaking the habit

In January 1933, two clinicians at the New York State Psychiatric Institute received an unusual proposition. Siegfried Katz and Carney Landis were visited by a twenty-four-year-old man (referred to as Z by Katz and Landis) who theorised that sleep was merely a habit – and a habit that he could break. Z suggested an experiment, to be overseen by Katz and Landis, in which he would endeavour to go without sleep for more than a week. Z hypothesised that 'at some time after a week of abstinence from sleep he would get a "second breath," and from that time on would be able to stay awake twenty-four hours a day without difficulty or effort'. In doing so, he would be benefiting 'the human race, since it would add at least a third more time to the life of every one who would go to the trouble of breaking the habit of sleep as he proposed to do'. With some misgivings, Katz and Landis bit and Z duly began his long sojourn in sleeplessness.

To test whether he was awake, the psychiatrists issued Z with a 'watchman's recording clock and key'. Z was instructed to turn the key every ten minutes, thereby punching a time stamp onto a paper strip in the clock. At regular intervals during the ten-day experiment – during which Z spent just five and a quarter hours napping – Katz and Landis performed a panoply of physiological and psychological tests. Some of these tests fell by the wayside. An assessment of Z's typing ability had to be abandoned on the fifth day. It hurt his eyes too much to focus on the paper.

According to Katz and Landis, Z never complained of tiredness. But by the third day he was experiencing hallucinations: of a cottage by the beach, an old man in a bathtub, or a whale. By the sixth day, disorientation had set in. He mistook a desk for a drinking fountain, for example, and forgot where he was. Z became increasingly irritable and argumentative – and paranoid. In fact, his paranoia was the chief reason why the experiment was ended after 231 hours:

During the course of the vigil Z formulated a delusional system, attributing persecutory intent to one of the experimenters. He became more and more certain that this experimenter was personally interested in making life disagreeable for him and in interpreting his behavior in terms of pathologic mental mechanisms. These tendencies became so marked during the last two days of the vigil that they formed the principal basis for our decision to discontinue the experiment when we did. His protests and misinterpretations of motives and conduct became increasingly marked to an extent which made him more and more unmanageable and occupied more and more time and attention of all connected with the experimental laboratory. Six months after the end of the experiment

Z still retained part of the system of ideas concerning this fancied persecution.

What enticed Katz and Landis to undertake the experiment was the opportunity to test the idea that extended periods of sleeplessness could cause mental and physical damage: 'There are, however, no actually observed cases recorded in the medical literature which clearly indicate that extended vigils produce either mental disease or death.' The 'somewhat eccentric' Z was their self-selected guinea pig. What they observed seemed to them to suggest that this theory – and the anecdotal evidence on which it was based – was mistaken. Though noting that Z's 'higher functions of organisation and synthesis of mental life appeared to be somewhat affected', and that Z was still manifesting paranoia six months later, Katz and Landis nonetheless declared:

> It has been demonstrated that in this case it was possible to go with practically no sleep for approximately ten days without any known physiologic effect and without any permanent change in the personality or in the mental function. . . . Every change [in Z] which we have remarked on can in a way be reasonably viewed and explained on the basis of the general personality and character of the subject.

Arriving at such a conclusion necessitated a little selective blindness, of course. We don't know how long Z's paranoia lasted, but I would certainly call it a significant change to mental function. That Katz and Landis did not may tell us something about the importance, or lack of it, attached to paranoid thoughts back then. Or perhaps they considered Z to have been prone to paranoia all along (though if this was the case, they didn't say so).

Today we know much more about the importance of sleep, and the unhappy consequences of not getting enough of it. That's why Katz and Landis's experiment would not be permissible today. One day someone may break the world record of 265 hours without sleep set by Californian high-school student Randy Gardner in 1964. But their name won't be listed by Guinness. Prolonged sleeplessness is too dangerous to encourage. Physically, sleep loss has been linked to increased risk of stroke, Alzheimer's disease, chronic pain, cancer, diabetes, heart attacks, infertility, weight gain, obesity, and reduced immune response. Yet the significance of sleep in regard to psychological wellbeing is still underestimated, if not by patients then by many mental health professionals. When sleep issues occur alongside other psychological problems, the tendency has been to see them primarily as a consequence of those other difficulties. As such, it's assumed that they don't need to be treated in their own right. Deal with the primary disorder – depression, anxiety or psychosis, for example – and the patient will sleep like a baby again. (It took until publication of the fifth edition of the *Diagnostic and Statistical Manual* in 2013 for the American Psychiatric Association to recommend that 'secondary' sleep problems be diagnosed and treated as independent disorders.)

We were given a revealing insight into clinical attitudes to sleep when Aliyah Rehman, Andrew Gumley and colleagues in Glasgow and my team surveyed staff treating psychosis patients in Glasgow and Oxfordshire. One hundred and eleven people participated, mostly psychiatric nurses and psychiatrists, but also some psychologists, occupational therapists and social workers. Everyone reported sleep problems in their patients, usually insomnia (difficulty falling and staying asleep) and hypersomnia (oversleeping). They knew that these issues made it much harder for patients to function effectively during the day. And, encouragingly, almost everyone thought that poor sleep and psychotic symptoms fed off each other, rather than the former simply following on from the latter.

But when it came to assessing and treating sleep problems, things weren't so positive. Few clinicians used formal methods of assessment. They generally just asked their patients how they were sleeping. Now, that's a perfectly good starting place. But it's not the most effective way of pinpointing what's going on, nor of measuring how things might be changing. (It was not unknown in the past for psychosis patients' complaints of being up all night to be dismissed as exaggeration. The advent of activity monitors has shown that these patients' accounts are often entirely accurate.) As for treatment, most clinicians used medication and/or advice on what's called 'sleep hygiene'. Sleep hygiene techniques (ensuring your bedroom is quiet and comfortable, for instance, or avoiding daytime naps) can be useful for many people, but on their own they don't tend to be effective for treating insomnia. Very few clinicians provided the cognitive behavioural therapies that the National Institute for Health and Care Excellence (NICE) recommends and that can be so effective for sleep disorders.

'I'm going to fall asleep here'

'I used to stay in bed trying to get some sleep for hours, things going through my mind. I used to wake up in the middle of the night and I used to get up very early in the morning as well.'

When I began investigating the relationship between sleep and paranoia back in 2008, it seemed to some a strange move. Indeed, a senior colleague at the Institute of Psychiatry warned that it could be a career-defining step (and not in a good way). 'You don't want to be doing all that non-specific stuff,' I was advised. In other words, focus on a particular disorder, rather than a difficulty that cuts across disorders and defines none. I knew very little about sleep problems. Even today they are given scant attention in clinical training programmes. But so many patients were telling me about their sleep difficulties that this 'non-specific stuff' seemed much more significant than that.

I was in no doubt that poor sleep was causing real distress and exacerbating other psychological problems. Patients reported crushing fatigue: 'I was shattered all the time.' One patient was so exhausted that they warned, right in the middle of a consultation, 'I'm going to fall asleep here.' Insomnia was wreaking havoc with their mood: 'I am more nervous and worried if I don't get sleep'; 'I was stroppy all the time'; 'I'm more agitated if I haven't slept for two or three days'. And it was preventing people from getting on with normal activities: 'It annoyed me, because I was just wasting time really being asleep all day'; 'It wasn't giving me enough time to do what I wanted during the day'; 'it was affecting my social life'. In a nutshell: 'When I'm tired, everything is worse'.

I began by trying to establish whether what I saw in clinic was truly representative. How common were sleep problems in people with persecutory delusions? And what about the general population: was there an association between insomnia and everyday paranoia? To find out, I recruited thirty patients being treated at the Maudsley Hospital, and three hundred local adults without a history of severe mental health disorder. As is often the way with early-stage research, there was no funding. So I tagged it on to other studies, collecting additional data to help decide whether I was on to something or not. It was not a surprise to discover that a large majority of the patient group (83 per cent) were getting insufficient sleep. Over 50 per cent reported clinical levels of insomnia and in more than half of those cases the problem was at the top end of the severity scale. And the community group? Almost 30 per cent had symptoms of insomnia, with around 10 per cent scoring highly enough to indicate a possible clinical disorder. Moreover, the link between sleep problems and paranoia was unmistakeable. When I looked, for example, at the scores of those with the highest levels of mistrust, 60 per cent were above the threshold for clinical insomnia. In stark contrast, hardly any of those with the lowest paranoia scores reported significant sleep problems (just 8 per cent). Higher levels of insomnia meant higher levels of paranoia – probably because of the negative effect sleep problems have on mood.

A very similar picture emerged when I analysed data from the 2007 British Adult Psychiatric Morbidity Survey. As we saw in Chapter 4, the APMS isn't focused on people with mental health problems but instead covers a representative sample of 8,580 members of the English general public. It turned out that paranoia was at least twice as likely to occur in people with insomnia. And the worse the insomnia, the more severe the paranoia. The 6.6 per cent with chronic insomnia, for instance, were five times more likely to report that there had been times when they believed a group of people was plotting to cause them serious harm. It's the same story internationally. The World Health Organization's mammoth World Health Survey, carried out between 2002 and 2004, included 260,000 adults from seventy countries across the globe from India to Ivory Coast, Denmark to the Dominican Republic. On average, people with sleep problems were twice as likely to report paranoid thoughts.

I was pretty sure that this wasn't a coincidence, although with one-off studies like these one can't be certain. But my hunch that sleep problems might be actually *causing* mistrust was given a boost when I looked at responses to the first APMS.

The initial round of interviews for that survey took place in 2000, with a subset of 2,382 participants assessed again eighteen months later. That allows us to see how things changed, and to infer – on the basis of hard data rather than supposition – what might lie behind those changes. Insomnia proved to be the strongest predictor of subsequent paranoia (alongside worry, which we'll get to in Chapter 11). Indeed, people who reported insomnia at their first assessment had 3.5 times the chance of later developing paranoia compared to those who had not.

My APMS work was the first longitudinal study of paranoia and insomnia – that's to say, the first analysis of their incidence and relationship over time. The results weren't proof of a causal link. But they strengthened my conviction that, if we could help patients with their sleep problems, it would be a lot easier to tackle their paranoia (and indeed other psychological problems they might be experiencing). We had to listen to what patients were telling us about this 'non-specific stuff' – and act upon it.

From BEST to the OASIS

Sleep problems are extremely common. On any given night, one in three people will be struggling. Around 10 per cent of adults have experienced clinical levels of insomnia in the previous twelve months. And in my 2023 survey of 10,000 UK adults, around 20–25 per cent of people reported significant problems sleeping over the previous fortnight. (By now you won't be surprised to learn that this group was also more prone to mistrust.) The good news is that there is a very effective treatment: CBT-I, or cognitive behavioural therapy for insomnia. The bad news for people with persecutory delusions, as we have seen, is that next to no one is offered CBT-I. But as recently as

2015, the situation was worse because no one had even properly
tested CBT-I for psychosis patients.

It was high time for us to do something about it. We recruited
fifty people with long-standing insomnia and persecutory delusions to what we called the Better Sleep Trial or, because
scientists love an acronym, BEST. As is inevitably the case with
diagnostic labels, the term insomnia can only hint at the
complexity, diversity and sheer misery of the problems experienced by the people in our study. Some patients were going to
bed early in the evening and then lying awake for hours. Some
were only heading to bed in the early hours of the morning.
Some associated bed with past trauma. And some didn't even
have a bed. Patients were awake and pacing all night. For some
patients the hypnotic medication prescribed to treat their
insomnia just made things worse. They were perpetually drowsy
and napping throughout the day. Their sleep, in other words,
was a mess.

Half of the participants – the control group – continued with
standard care. That comprised antipsychotic medication and
contact with the clinical team, but little or nothing directly
targeting their sleep problems. The others received standard
care plus our sleep therapy, delivered in eight one-to-one sessions
with a clinical psychologist. We tweaked the contents of that
therapy in line with the requirements of the individual participant. But four features were key. The first was circadian
realignment, which involves sorting out the daily routine. That
means gradually making sure people are going to bed and
waking up at the right times and eating regular meals. The
second was stimulus control. The objective is to learn to associate bed with sleep, rather than with watching TV or eating
or working. If sleep isn't happening, you get out of bed. Third
was reducing night-time anxiety and arousal by implementing
a relaxing wind-down routine and reducing caffeine use in the

later part of the day. Lastly, we built up the pressure for sleep by increasing activity levels during the day.

Eight sessions. Eight hours of contact time with a therapist. That was all it took for many of our patients to experience much better sleep. Checking in twelve weeks after beginning the sleep intervention, nine of the twenty-five (41 per cent) no longer had insomnia. Benefits were still there when we assessed the patients after twenty-four weeks. Patients felt much less fatigue and much greater psychological wellbeing. But if the therapy produced large clinical improvements in sleep, what did it do to paranoia? It looked as though better sleep brought modest reductions in mistrust, but the trial was too small for us to be sure. What we needed was a really large study. So I roped in clinical psychologists from across the UK. And I drafted in expertise from the newly founded Oxford Sleep and Circadian Neurosciences Institute led by Professor Russell Foster, a pioneer in the neurobiology of circadian rhythms and (I was rather envious to discover) a trustee of London's Science Museum. Together we conducted the biggest ever randomised controlled trial of a psychological intervention for a mental health problem.

Beginning in March 2015, we recruited 3,755 students with insomnia from twenty-six UK universities. Half were randomly assigned to a digital CBT sleep therapy program called Sleepio (the brainchild of the clinical psychologist Colin Espie). Sleepio is made up of six weekly web-based sessions, each lasting an average of twenty minutes. The other half of the group received care as normal, which in most cases meant little or no treatment for insomnia. This was the Oxford Access for Students Improving Sleep study – or, adding to our acronym collection, OASIS. We followed the students for twenty-two weeks. And we discovered that, sure enough, treating insomnia didn't just bring large improvements in sleep, it reduced rates of paranoia too. Those reductions were small, but they were significant and sustained.

The sleep therapy also resulted in fewer cases of hallucinations, nightmares, depression and anxiety, and boosted general psychological wellbeing. OASIS nailed, once and I hope for all, the idea that poor sleep is merely a by-product of mental health problems. On the contrary, sleep issues can play a major role in *causing* those problems. And then the two make each other worse. On the flipside, OASIS – and BEST before it – show just how much there is to be gained by treating sleep problems seriously, no matter what other difficulties the individual may also be grappling with.

For one thing, it could lead to people spending less time in psychiatric hospital. This is clearly desirable for patients, but it is also a boon for the public purse. In-patient care swallows almost 20 per cent of the UK's budget for adult mental health. Even with this expenditure there is acute pressure on beds: the average ward runs above capacity. That means patients often having to be hospitalised many miles from home. We know that there is a correlation between patients' sleep problems on admission and duration of hospitalisation. Given what we've seen in this chapter about the relationship between sleep and mental health, that is no surprise. Unfortunately, psychiatric wards tend not to be conducive to good sleep. They can be noisy; lights often need to be switched on periodically through the night so that staff can observe patients; and there may not be much natural daylight, further disrupting already unsettled body clocks.

Alvaro Barrera, a wonderful psychiatrist who leads an in-patient ward in Oxford, had been in touch to ask whether I could offer his patients psychological therapies. He gave me a tour of the ward, and I was struck by how warmly he was greeted by patients and staff alike. What better place, I thought, to see whether our sleep research could help in-patients? And Bryony Sheaves got to work, ably supported by Louise Isham and Josie McInerney (our team's resident American footballer). We piloted a two-week CBT treatment for insomnia with patients newly admitted to the ward, which treats adult men. Most of the patients are admitted during an acute episode of psychosis or bipolar disorder, and each of them has their own bedroom. The treatment was structured around three principal strategies. First, we encouraged patients to be more active during the day – and thus more tired at bedtime. Next, we worked on establishing a proper bedtime wind-down routine. When you've just been detained in a psychiatric ward, and are experiencing distressing psychological changes, becoming sufficiently calm to even contemplate sleep is often a very big ask. Lastly, we tried to reinforce the psychological link between bed and sleep.

But the setting necessitated some creative thinking. It's difficult, for instance, for a patient to only use their bed for sleeping when they have no other private space – and when, for patients with persecutory delusions, the ward's communal spaces can feel like no-go areas. And even for those individuals who aren't fearful of staff or other patients, the hubbub of the brightly lit ward doesn't lend itself to a relaxing night-time wind down. So, we equipped patients' rooms with a beanbag. It may not sound like much, but it gave people a comfortable, quiet place to spend time. And it meant they could reserve their bed for sleep. To help create a restful environment, we supplied eye masks and blackout curtains, recorded relaxation exercises and downloaded restful music onto a USB stick, and brought in battery-operated radios on which to play them (power cables weren't an option given that they could be used as a ligature). To help patients be more alert and active during the day we worked with the ward staff to organise walks in the hospital garden or the local park. Napping is a major disruptor of sleep on the ward, partly because people are often bored and partly because their illness and/or medication fatigues them.

So we scheduled these walks for times when the individual might ordinarily be tempted to nap. For people who were too unwell to leave the ward – or who were not permitted to do so – we supplied light boxes, administering 10,000 lux of light for thirty minutes at a time. (Ten thousand lux is equivalent to natural daylight – which is critical for our sleep–wake cycle. By contrast, the artificial light in which patients usually spend their time is only around 100–300 lux.) And we set gradually increasing step counts – and provided an activity tracking watch to measure progress.

Psychiatric wards can be challenging environments for research, but the treatment proved highly effective in treating patients' insomnia – and it led to them leaving hospital eight and a half days earlier than individuals who hadn't received it. Is this enormously encouraging result generalisable? That remains to be seen. We haven't yet managed to secure funding to test the intervention at scale on hospital wards.

Treating sleep problems may even help prevent people developing psychosis. Problems typically begin during adolescence with 'psychotic-like experiences'. These are less intense or frequent versions of the sort of difficulties – including paranoia – seen in psychosis proper. Psychotic-like experiences often follow periods of poor sleep, which also makes them more likely to persist and to develop into a clinical disorder. There are plenty of reasons, therefore, to take sleep problems seriously in this group. Yet research has been sparse. In fact, no one had trialled a treatment until, with Jonathan Bradley and Felicity Waite carrying out the work, we did so in 2017. Our pilot involved eleven participants aged fifteen to twenty-two. All were in contact with mental health services and considered at ultra-high risk of severe mental health problems. (Around 20 per cent of young people in this category go on to develop psychosis.) It's worth noting where these young people were starting from:

'I would just sleep through the day and that like put a massive strain on like my social aspect and mood and my mental health, and I just think that it just turned my life like the other way around, so I would be up at night and then, because I was up at night, I wouldn't be up in the day and I wouldn't go out and see people because I was sleeping, and it was just . . . I just think it was very unhealthy.'

'. . . not being able to get to sleep, not being able to stay asleep, and then being too tired during the day to actually do anything, which was really, really affecting my mood.'

From this inauspicious base, we saw really encouraging improvements in sleep after the eight-session treatment. Six of the group no longer met the criteria for clinical insomnia and nine had fallen below the threshold for sleep problems we'd used when recruiting participants. Levels of anxiety and depression declined, and the group reported significant reductions in paranoia and other psychotic experiences:

'. . . the stuff that I normally wouldn't have done because I was physically just too tired, I find I can now have the energy to do that, those things, which makes me feel happy because I'm getting stuff done and I'm not getting stressed out at the fact that I haven't done the things that I wanted to do. It makes me feel happier.'

'. . . the depression has been the big step. It's really eased. It's nowhere near where it used to be.'

'I find it also has helped my anxiety a lot. I'm able to cope with situations a lot better and kind of stay in control, which I think has come from me gaining control of my sleep a bit.'

Led by Felicity Waite, we've recently tested the therapy – now named SleepWell – in a randomised controlled trial with forty young people in contact with mental health services and at ultra-high risk of psychosis. SleepWell made good on the promise of the pilot, delivering substantial improvements in the participants' sleep. And when we checked in with the group nine months after treatment they were still sleeping better. There were additional benefits: rates of depression, anxiety and paranoia all fell during treatment (and had fallen even further at follow-up). Given that the participants had reported levels of paranoia comparable to what we see in patients with a psychosis diagnosis, the transformation seemed especially remarkable. We need a bigger trial, for sure, and Felicity is leading that now. But the signs so far are enormously encouraging.

Sleep deprivation revisited

One way of demonstrating the importance of sleep to mental health is to treat insomnia and see how that affects wellbeing. The other, of course, is to restrict sleep. This is what Katz and Landis had done in 1933, and what Sarah Reeve, Bryony Sheaves and I did some eighty-five years later. We recruited seventy-five young people from Oxford, all of whom enjoyed trouble-free sleep – until they fell into Sarah's clutches, at any rate. All were in good psychological shape, with no history of psychiatric problems. For three days our volunteers were requested simply to follow their normal sleep pattern. On average, that amounted to approximately seven hours sleep a night. It must have seemed like an easy gig. But another week (either preceding or following) we asked them to delay their bedtime, allowing a maximum of four hours of sleep for three consecutive nights. Someone who normally slept from 11 p.m. to 7 a.m., for instance, would now have to make do with sleeping from 3 a.m. to 7 a.m. To check whether they'd fallen asleep, we asked them to reply to hourly text messages. And they wore motion-detecting devices so that we could monitor their movement.

It couldn't have been much fun – though at least, I suppose, we weren't suggesting anyone replicate Z's epic ten days of sleeplessness. But their efforts were not in vain: the results were striking. Among the group overall, going without sleep produced an increase in paranoia (measured using the Specific Psychotic Experiences Questionnaire). It also sparked hallucination-like experiences and cognitive confusion; like paranoia, the latter are often seen in patients with psychosis. Moreover, these experiences caused a lot more distress than they did when people had slept well. As if all this were not enough, three days of sleep deprivation was sufficient to trigger symptoms of depression, anxiety and worry. As you were doubtless told as a child: never underestimate the importance of a good night's sleep.

Hypersomnia and nightmares

'I don't want nine hours sleep. Your life's boring enough without sleeping too much.'

Insomnia tends to be the most common sleep problem in patients with persecutory delusions, just as it is the most prevalent generally. But it certainly isn't the only one. When Sarah Reeve (who may own to liking her sleep) assessed sixty patients being treated for their first episode of psychosis, almost a quarter reported excessive sleepiness. This sleepiness, combined with regularly sleeping for more than nine hours a night or for more than eleven hours during a twenty-four-hour period, is termed hypersomnia – and 71 per cent of the clinicians surveyed by

Aliyah Rehman listed it as one of the sleep problems they saw most often in patients.

Hypersomnia is often assumed to be simply a consequence of taking antipsychotic drugs. There is no disputing the impact of medication. In one international patient survey, feeling sleepy during the day was reported as the number one side effect of antipsychotics, experienced by 83 per cent of the respondents. (That said, the picture is a complex one. For a patient who is struggling to sleep at night, the sedative properties of antipsychotics can be helpful. But the timing and quantity of the dose has to be spot on. Get it wrong and people are still groggy in the daytime. It can be a difficult balance to strike.) Nevertheless, Sarah's analysis suggested that there is more to hypersomnia than the effects of medication. Inactivity might be a factor, possibly because people are spending a lot more time in bed. Influential too may be other sleep problems: insomnia, nightmares, and sleep-related movement disorders like restless leg syndrome (unbearable discomfort in the legs, which can only be relieved by moving them). In other words, people are oversleeping because they are so shattered by previous broken nights.

Patients also often complain of repeated nightmares. Exactly how common they are in this group isn't clear: we still await definitive studies. But estimates range from 9 per cent to 55 per cent of patients. (In the general population the figure is probably somewhere between 2 and 8 per cent.) Nightmares don't merely exhaust people, they cause really significant distress. Indeed, experiencing frequent nightmares raises the risk of suicidal ideation and death by suicide, both among those with a psychosis diagnosis and in the general population. Nightmares may play a special role in paranoia – perhaps by presenting us with an image of the harm we fear, perhaps because of their negative effect on our emotions, or quite possibly both. For all this, nightmares are almost never assessed or treated when people come to services.

So Bryony Sheaves decided to try a brief CBT intervention. At the core of that intervention was the standard technique for treating nightmares: imagery rescripting (IR). Essentially, IR involves reshaping the story of your nightmare, changing it in any way you like, and spending a little time each day running through the new version in your mind. The trial – a pilot with twenty-four patients, half of whom received the treatment from Bryony – was the first of its kind. No one had tested this kind of therapy with this patient group, which tells its own story about attitudes to sleep problems in mental health care. The results underlined the scale of the oversight. Bryony saw a sizeable reduction in the severity of nightmares, on a par with what IR produces in people without psychosis. The intervention also brought about a big improvement in insomnia. As we've seen throughout this chapter, if we can improve sleep, we're likely to have a positive effect on paranoia. And that's what happened here. As the participants' nightmares receded, their persecutory delusions began to do likewise.

* * *

Who would have guessed it? The 'non-specific stuff' turns out to be a major influence on psychological wellbeing. Sleeping poorly lowers our mood, raises our anxiety levels – and breeds paranoia. Not only are sleep disorders common, there is growing concern that many of us without clinical insomnia are sleeping much less than is healthy. (Whether or not we're sleeping less than in the past is a matter of debate, but on balance things don't seem to have changed much over the last sixty years.) The US Centers for Disease Control and Prevention (CDC) notes that almost 15 per cent of adults struggle to fall asleep most nights and nearly 18 per cent have trouble staying asleep. Adults typically require between seven and nine hours sleep a night, but the CDC data suggests almost 30 per cent of people don't reach the minimum. Could this endemic sleeplessness spawn an upsurge in mistrust?

8.

All the rubbish that you are

'Saying it to you now sounds daft, but at the time it was like I had a life bailiff at the door going: "Right, come on. Answer for yourself. What have you been up to? Why are you off sick? Why are you doing this, why are you doing that?" Now I know it was a figment of my imagination but at the time it was real.'

'Who did you think was going to call you to account?'

'I thought about the people in my life I was accountable to, like my boss. And I was a teacher, so the students in my class. My parents as well – I should explain myself. A shopkeeper who I'd dealt with years ago. And they all kind of merged into one as one giant force of "answer for yourself".'

'How did this play out day to day?'

'I didn't really want to look out of the window because I thought I would see people looking into the house. It must sound crazy . . . Almost like spies. "Has she got up yet? Has she done any exercise? Has she had her breakfast?" – because I was starving myself at the time. So, I wouldn't go close to the window, which sounds so strange, I know. And thinking that every email and every call and every number I didn't recognise was somebody coming to get me.

'I could very easily be my own worst critic. I could look at the absolute minutiae of myself and the decisions I'd made and the words I'd said, the things I'd written or the places I'd been.

And I had a lot of time to ruminate over it. To go through it with a fine toothcomb. And if anyone's going to catch me out it's going to be me. And I was very comfortable being ruthless with myself – finding my flaws. And if you sit for a long time, you'll find some negative stuff on yourself. It's almost like collating an invisible list. Right: let's put down all the rubbish that you are. And it became so natural.'

'Why did you do that?'

'I don't know if it goes to me perhaps choosing to go against the grain with the decisions I've made in my life. I was the first one to go to university. I was the first one to go outside of Europe or to work abroad, or to have two boyfriends instead of one and marrying him. So I was going against the grain from dot really. So maybe that accountability on myself goes back to being young and it became a habit.'

'You were always a little self-critical?'

'That's very kind of you to say a little bit! No: I was incredibly self-critical. But ever so kind to other people, and reasonable, and logical, and generally lovely and understanding. But an absolute nightmare to myself.'

'When you'd withdrawn into your room and these ideas had really taken hold, what were the signs that actually you were being observed and that there might be a reckoning coming?'

'If for example I got an email from my boss saying: "When are you coming back?" That is legitimate, that did happen, but then I'd think that supports my theory that everyone is after me. And my work is after me. No: your work is just asking when are you coming back because they need to sort out your visa. What a powerful imagination I had!'

Paranoia and self-esteem

All the rubbish that you are. Cherry's words have stayed with me, though our conversation is now several years in the past. They sum up so well, and so movingly, the feelings of most of the patients I meet. Like Cherry at her lowest, their sense of themselves is extremely negative. They believe they are different from, and inferior to, other people. They are, like Cherry, their 'own worst critics'. What I have observed in clinical practice has been borne out by numerous studies. In fact, it was the subject of my first ever paper, published in 1998, when I found that almost three-quarters of patients with persecutory delusions reported very low self-esteem. We know too that the lower a person's self-esteem, the more troubling and persistent their paranoia. This no doubt explains why the wellbeing of people with persecutory delusions – the severest form of paranoia – is often on the floor, with around half of psychosis patients scoring among the lowest 2 per cent in the population. Sadly, the combination of debilitating paranoia and rock-bottom self-esteem is potentially lethal. In 2019 I surveyed 110 patients with persistent persecutory delusions. Around three-quarters had contemplated killing themselves in the previous month. Around two-thirds experienced these thoughts ('suicidal ideation') at least weekly. Surveys of the general population suggest that approximately one in ten people will ponder suicide at some stage. But for patients with persecutory delusions, suicidal ideation isn't confined to a small minority. It is the norm.

What do we mean by low self-esteem? Which specific self-beliefs do people with paranoia typically endorse? In 2006 David Fowler and I devised a new questionnaire, the Brief Core Schema Scale (BCSS). The scale included six negative statements about the self:

- I am unloved.
- I am worthless.
- I am weak.
- I am vulnerable.
- I am bad.
- I am a failure.

Since David and I put together the BCSS, study after study has shown that people who agree with these statements are more likely to be paranoid. This is true not only for those being treated in mental health services, but among the general population too. And these negative ideas about the self don't just sit alongside paranoid thoughts: they predict them. For patients with persecutory delusions, the lower their self-esteem the more likely it is that their paranoia will persist. Among the general population, low self-esteem doubles the odds of later paranoia.

'I just think I'm ugly'

With work led by Felicity Waite in my research group, a new perspective on these negative self-beliefs has recently opened up. How we feel about ourselves is of course a complex business, the product of multiple interacting factors. Frequently, one of those factors is physical appearance. Ours is a culture, after all, that attaches huge significance to how we look – as pretty much everyone recognises. A 2021 YouGov survey, for example, found that almost 90 per cent of people in the UK believe that physical appearance matters, either a great deal (46 per cent) or somewhat (43 per cent). And 87 per cent agreed that good-looking people fare better in life because of their appearance. (Broadly speaking, research tends to suggest that this is true.) It's a little surprising then that the impact of body image on the self-esteem of people with persecutory delusions has been overlooked. In my experience patients are often concerned about their weight and that feeds into a sense of social vulnerability. The message came over loud and clear when Emily Marshall, a doctoral student supervised by Felicity and myself, interviewed twelve patients in 2020:

'I'm just not happy with the way I am, what I look like, what I look like to other people.' (Echo)

'I'm depressed most of the time. I'm angry with myself that I'm overweight. I don't like being overweight. And every time I go to Slimming World, and I haven't lost very much, I get angry with myself.' (John)

One of the factors dragging down the self-esteem of the people we spoke to was the medication they had been prescribed. Antipsychotics often trigger rapid weight gain:

'I ballooned up to twenty-three stone.' (Echo)

'I couldn't recognise myself hardly.' (Hillary)

'Yeah, I think it's hard with the medications because you're trying really hard to diet but then your medication is making you crave food and you're sort of in a constant battle to try and diet and you just can't do it because the medication's making you crave the food.' (Percy)

Ballooning to twenty-three stone is distressing enough, but to do so in a society in which obesity is highly stigmatised only increases the psychological toll on patients. As the psychologists Rebecca Puhl and Chelsea Heuer have noted: 'Weight bias translates into inequities in employment settings, health-care facilities, and educational institutions, often due to widespread negative

stereotypes that overweight and obese persons are lazy, unmo-
tivated, lacking in self-discipline, less competent, noncompliant,
and sloppy.' (Yes, you read that correctly: we're not talking
name-calling by ignorant kids but rather entrenched and consequential prejudice from employers, healthcare professionals and
teachers, among many others.)

Many of the participants told Emily that worries about their
appearance directly fuelled their paranoia:

> 'They're talking about me . . . they're judging me from how
> I look.' (Percy)

> 'It's the people walking past me or behind me. I have a fear
> of men walking behind me. I feel they are laughing at me
> and, you know, they're gonna get to me and it's horrible.'

> *'Why do you think they might be laughing at you?'*

> 'I don't know, it's the way I probably look.' (Mandy)

Once again, what we see here with patients isn't an anomaly.
When Felicity and I looked at data on the US general population
we saw a similar picture. In both the National Comorbidity
Survey – Replication (NCS-R) and the NCS-R's Adolescent
Supplement (NCS-A), participants were asked: 'Was there ever
a time in your life when you had a great deal of concern about/
worried a great deal or strongly feared being too fat or overweight?' Those who answered yes to this question – over 35 per
cent of the adults and 28 per cent of the adolescents – were
much more likely to report paranoid thoughts.

Height, self-esteem and paranoia: A VR investigation

'You are younger, and yet, I'll be bound, you are taller and
twice as broad across the shoulders; you could knock him
down in a twinkling; don't you feel that you could?'
                    Emily Brontë, *Wuthering Heights* (1847)

'I want to know what's the point? I'm paying taxes for this
lot to study height . . .'
                    Paul Daniels, magician and television presenter

A pathway from negative ideas about oneself to paranoia made
theoretical sense. Paranoia feeds on a sense of personal vulnerability. Believing that you're weak or worthless or unattractive
is likely to fuel that idea of vulnerability. The data we'd gathered
until then seemed to back up this idea. But to be certain we
needed a different kind of evidence. If you really want to prove
that something affects something else, you need to carry out a
causal test. That means manipulating one variable and measuring the effect on another. So I wanted to see what happened
if we made someone feel more negatively about themselves.
Would they become more likely to experience paranoia?
Conversely, could we reduce mistrust by boosting self-esteem?
I began to plan an unusual experiment.

Most of us tend to exaggerate our height. Given the advantages conferred on the tall, this is unsurprising. Taller people
spend longer in full-time education and they are more likely to
hold a degree than shorter people with the same cognitive abil-
ities. They are more likely to work in professional or
managerial roles. A person who is six foot tall is likely to earn
around £135,000 more over the course of a thirty-year career
than someone who is five foot five. In fact, in the US, for every

inch of height a man is almost 10 per cent more likely to be employed in a high-status job than as a labourer (for women, the figure is 4.6 per cent). As if this weren't sufficient, being tall is likely to help your romantic life too. As the Italian proverb puts it: *altezza mezza bellezza* (height is half of beauty). Taller adolescents of both sexes typically date more than their shorter peers. Tall men are more likely to find a long-term partner, or indeed several. And an analysis of 20,000 Italian couples found that taller people ended up with more educated, and more highly paid, partners.

Given that tall people appear to have the world at their feet, it is hardly surprising that they also enjoy certain psychological benefits. Height is associated with greater happiness and self-esteem, less pain and sadness, and a markedly reduced rate of suicide. Doubtless these psychological advantages stem in part from the pervasive tendency to associate height with power. Even babies as young as ten months are sensitive to social hier-archies, and they assume that size correlates with dominance. That tendency is embedded in our language. We 'look up' to people we consider superior. Those without influence are the 'little people'. Height is taken as an index of leadership ability. Among US Fortune 500 companies, the average CEO stands a little under six foot tall – around three inches taller than the average US man. Thirty per cent of these CEOs are six foot tall or more. Among the US population only 4 per cent of men are that tall. It is now more than 120 years since the United States elected a president who was shorter than the average American. William McKinley, victor in 1897, measured five foot seven and was duly ridiculed in the press as a 'little boy'. The same fate befell Napoleon Bonaparte, derided by the British as a ranting pipsqueak despite being two inches taller than the average contemporary Frenchman. In Bonaparte's case the mud has stuck via the theory of the Napoleon complex. This is the idea that short men compensate for their lack of stature with supercharged levels of determination, dominance and aggression. Moreover, we don't merely assume the tall are powerful. When we feel more commanding, we tend to overestimate our own height.

If height and self-esteem are so enmeshed, what are the psychological consequences of feeling smaller than usual? My hunch was that the experience would cause people to view themselves more negatively, reducing their sense of status and self-esteem, triggering a sense of vulnerability – and hence making them more mistrustful. How can someone experience the same situation from differing heights? In 1957 Sophia Loren was asked to stand in a trench while shooting *Boy on a Dolphin* so she didn't appear taller than her male co-star Alan Ladd. (Similar tricks are rumoured to be in use in today's entertainment business. Tom Cruise is thought to be one of the stars who have benefited.) Lacking a trench, I took a different tack: virtual reality.

The participants in my VR experiment were sixty women who had experienced paranoid thoughts in the previous month. (Being tall has advantages for both men and women, but there are minor differences, and so I decided to test a single-sex group.) None of the participants had a history of severe mental health problems. The volunteers took a six-minute ride on the simulated tube train I described in Chapter 4. During their time in the VR world, the sounds of a typical platform and tube journey – the rumble of the train, the hum of other passengers' conversations – were played through headphones. And as normal on the tube, there were plenty of other people around. In this case it was computer-generated avatars, all programmed to behave in a strictly neutral fashion.

The participants took the virtual tube journey twice: once at normal height and once with their perspective altered to mimic how the scene would look if they were about a head shorter. (The order of journeys was randomised: some people started with their height unchanged; others began in the meta-phorical trench.) The results were dramatic. When they were smaller, the participants were much more likely to feel inferior, weak and incompetent. Crucially, they were also more prone to paranoia, believing for example that someone in the carriage was being hostile or trying to upset them by staring. The data proved this wasn't a chance association. The increase in paranoia was fully accounted for by the increase in negative thoughts about the self.

We didn't tell the participants that we had reduced their height, and almost no one noticed. 'It felt different in the two times. I felt more vulnerable the first time, and also the man with the legs in the aisle was acting in a hostile way towards me the first time, but I didn't feel it so much the second time, even though his legs were in the same place, I don't know why!' was a typical comment. Another participant remarked: 'I felt more intimidated the first time, not sure why. There was a girl who kept putting her hand to her face, the man with the blue T-shirt was shaking his head at me, they were staring more at me.'

I was excited by these results. For the first time we had proof that negative thoughts about the self are a cause of paranoia. The resulting academic article drew a lot of media attention. But I must admit that some of the coverage was not entirely positive. The study was often misinterpreted as asserting that short people are more likely to be paranoid or that 'short man syndrome' is a reality. It showed neither of these things, of course, but I still receive emails from people explaining that, though they are not tall, neither are they paranoid. Shorter celebrities were summoned to defend their stature. The late magician Paul Daniels (five foot five) appeared on BBC Radio 4's

World at One show to decry a study that could be of value only to 'the virtual people of the world'. Daniels' catchphrase – 'You'll like this . . . not a lot, but you'll like it!' – clearly didn't extend to my work. Shortly before going on air on another station, I was taken aback by the news that I was going to be discussing my experiment with Wee Jimmy Krankie (international readers may want to pause here to consult the internet). My memory of the subsequent interview is hazy, but I think Wee Jimmy was more receptive to my thinking than the producers may have expected.

A glutton for punishment, I followed up the experiment a couple of years later, this time working with Stephanie Atherton, an Oxford psychology undergraduate. Stephanie recruited twenty-six men for the study. Again, none were psychiatric patients, though all had recently experienced paranoid thoughts. Just as the previous group had done, the participants rode the virtual tube train twice. Rather than altering their height, however, we prefaced each ride with an exercise designed either to boost or lower self-esteem. So Stephanie invited participants to explore a time when their self-confidence was at its peak. *Imagine that you'd been invited to a gathering back then, and you'd spent a while talking to a stranger. How would you have felt? What did you make of the person you chatted to? And what do you think they'd have thought of you?* The other exercise was identical, save for the fact that participants focused on the moment of their lowest self-confidence.

Brief though they were, those exercises had a substantial impact on how the participants perceived their virtual tube rides:

'It's funny, because I didn't think people in virtual reality could ever really appear hostile, or like they intended to cause me harm. But in the second one [low self-confidence], I definitely did notice people looking at me in that way.'

'I felt like I was being awkward the first time [low self-confidence], and that the guy opposite me was looking at me a bit, but the second time [high self-confidence] he looked more awkward.'

Taking that train journey with higher or lower self-confidence had a profound effect on the way participants interpreted their VR experience. Think of self-confidence as a set of weighing scales. Tip them into the negative and, as Stephanie and I saw, suspicion results.

'I think I am more confident. . .': Pilot therapies

If low self-esteem can make us susceptible to mistrust, cultivating a kinder view of ourselves should in theory counteract that paranoia. As ever, though, formulating a hypothesis is one thing. Proving it is quite another. I began by developing a six-session treatment using techniques from positive psychology. (Positive psychology was kickstarted in the 1990s by Martin Seligman at the University of Pennsylvania. Arguing that psychology had focused exclusively on mental ill health, Seligman called for 'the scientific study of positive human functioning and flourishing'. Thirty years later, it does look like positive psychology techniques are potentially helpful in ameliorating depression, anxiety and stress, and improving wellbeing and quality of life.)

The treatment was all about building optimistic, enthusiastic, generous beliefs about oneself – drowning out the carping of the inner critic with the supportive talk of a best friend. To achieve this, we focused on three areas. Number one: enabling patients to recognise their positive qualities. Ask them to describe their deficiencies and off they go: no problem. But identifying what's good about themselves? Often the response is total silence. They just can't think of anything. So we prompted them. We shared a long list of potential positive characteristics, going through them one by one, and reflecting together on their relevance. Gradually the individual becomes aware that they are, for instance, generous, kind and reliable. I can see it, and that helps them to see it too. Number two: encouraging the patient to play to their strengths. This means scheduling homework activities that utilise the positive qualities we've identified. Number three: switching attention to the positive by *savouring*. That means taking the time to notice every aspect of an experience, to bask in the sensation of the moment. As part of that effort, we asked the participants to keep a record of the pleasing things they'd experienced each day, no matter how small: a cup of coffee in the sunshine, a friendly chat, a favourite TV show.

In 2012–14 we piloted the treatment with patients from Oxford Health NHS Foundation Trust where I work. Sure enough, we saw significant increases in self-esteem. Participants felt much more content with themselves. What also occurred was a reduction in paranoia. That was enormously heartening, especially given that antipsychotic medication hadn't been able to shift the delusions. Pleasing too was the fact that patients really engaged with the techniques. People often drop out of trials. Indeed, they frequently abandon mental health treatment in general. But everyone completed the programme. They were keen to attend additional sessions. And, the ultimate yardstick, we received more thank you chocolates from patients than any study before or since:

'I thought it was excellent. My self-confidence has got better and I think more positively. Before, everything seemed like a really big problem and I worried a lot. I do still worry, but I tell myself I can't do anything about it so I write it down instead. I'm feeling really good at the moment.'

'I think I am more confident and I have a slightly different bearing. The way I feel in myself and the way I am in myself. . . . It really helped me to reverse the balance and swing the pendulum back. It's such a change to think about strengths after years of going to the doctors and saying what's wrong. I've started giving my doctor and care co-ordinator that I meet a copy of my CV with my education, work I've done and voluntary experience on. I tell them that this is the me that you don't see when I'm well.'

It was a small trial. Fifteen people received the therapy, while a control group continued with treatment as normal. But this pilot study convinced me that in self-esteem we had a lever we could pull to help people overcome paranoia. And so we included a module on boosting self-confidence in our Feeling Safe programme.

The compassionate coach

'It just brings a lot of love to myself and actually to believe that has been really nice.'

There are many ways to help someone feel more positively about themselves. The clinical psychologist Paul Gilbert has pioneered compassion-focused therapy, an approach that draws inspiration from Buddhist psychology: 'The healing properties of compassion have been written about for centuries. The Dalai Lama often stresses that if you want others to be happy – focus on compassion; if you want to be happy yourself – focus on compassion.'

But what exactly is self-compassion, and how can we increase it? Gilbert writes that 'self-compassion focuses on generating a particular type of emotion towards the self that can loosely be called self-warmth or self-kindness'. We recognise our suffering. We understand it as an inevitable part of what it means to be human. And we forgive ourselves. To develop this self-kindness, Gilbert recommends a range of techniques, one of which is the compassionate coach or perfect nurturer. We imagine a person who is there just for us, a source of comfort and support whenever we are troubled. The perfect nurturer cares deeply about us. They have our best interests at heart. And they instil in us the confidence that we can cope with life's challenges. Having created our compassionate coach, we can imagine how they would have helped us through a tricky situation in the past – and take them with us into similar situations in the future.

Could this work for patients with persistent persecutory delusions? And would it reduce their paranoia as well as raise their self-esteem? The first person to investigate was Ava Forkert, an excellent doctoral student supervised by Felicity Waite and myself. In 2020 Ava piloted a four-session treatment with twelve patients, meeting them individually twice a week for a fortnight. The intervention brought big improvements in the way people felt about themselves: 'I felt better in my skin . . . I've been having more positive self-talk with myself'; 'Since I've started doing it I've felt quite confident'; 'It just brings a lot of love to myself and actually to believe that has been really nice'. The participants weren't merely more comfortable with themselves. They felt more able to manage their problems: 'I'm looking at things different and not getting so wound up'; 'I'm better able to cope with things when they happen'; 'I've got control over my own brain'. Their paranoia duly declined too: 'I don't feel quite so threatened as I did. I feel a little bit safer, I would say, maybe a little less vulnerable'; 'I don't need to worry about anybody else and what they're thinking . . . I'm not as paranoid'.

Ava's findings were backed up by an experiment undertaken

by Poppy Brown, this time not with patients but with one hundred adults from the local population in Oxfordshire. All the participants experienced regular paranoid thoughts, but none had a history of severe mental health conditions. In four ten-minute sessions Poppy asked the volunteers to imagine their own compassionate coach, and to think through how that coach might help them in a demanding situation. After each session, participants stepped into virtual reality, in this case either an elevator or our London Underground train. Being surrounded by strangers – even our VR avatars, who you'll remember had been programmed to be strictly neutral in their behaviour and attitude – can be difficult for people inclined to paranoia. So these VR experiences were framed as an opportunity for participants to try out self-compassion, supported by their imaginary coach.

As we had hoped, the exercise really boosted people's kindness towards themselves. It also made a significant difference to levels of paranoia when compared to a control group. Here was another compelling demonstration of the way in which mistrust feeds on negative views about the self – and of what might be achieved therapeutically by targeting that malign influence. Self-compassion quietens the destructive voices: the ones constantly insinuating that we are weak and inadequate and thus an easy target for the malice of others.

The work we've looked at in this chapter – the epidemiological statistics, the experiments, the prototype therapies – confirms what patients with persecutory delusions have been telling clinicians for years: their self-esteem is often on the floor. More than this, it reveals that feeling badly about oneself isn't so much a consequence of paranoia (though it is that too). It is a *cause* of that mistrustfulness. This goes not just for those at the severest end of the paranoia spectrum, but for all points in between. Like genes, upbringing, trauma and sleep problems, low self-esteem is part of the mechanism of mistrust. In the next chapter we'll explore another: drugs.

* * *

All the rubbish that you are. Things have moved on for Cherry, who I got to know when she joined a panel of people with lived experience of mental health problems advising on my paranoia research. As I write this, she is throwing herself happily into the challenge of being a new mother while continuing to contribute to the research of myself and my team. She's getting along fine.

> I certainly didn't think little old me would have something of value to contribute, but it turns out perhaps I do . . . to think that in the future I would be contributing, I wouldn't have believed it. Just like I wouldn't have believed the way you're feeling isn't forever, and you are not your thoughts, and you will get better . . . I'm doing alright now.

9.

Why I'm quitting tobacco

In July 1798 Napoleon Bonaparte's Armée d'Orient conquered Egypt. Napoleon (who, as we learned in Chapter 8, was not the tiny man of English propaganda) was much taken with the country: 'In Egypt I found myself freed from the obstacles of an irksome civilisation. I was full of dreams. I saw myself founding a religion, marching into Asia, riding an elephant, a turban on my head and in my hand a new Koran that I would have composed to suit my need.' But Napoleon was dismayed by the local population's consumption of hashish, which had been the intoxicant of choice since its arrival from Asia during the Middle Ages. Even worse, his own soldiers took to this unfamiliar narcotic with gusto, no doubt partly because alcohol was impossible to come by in Islamic Egypt. Napoleon moved quickly to put an end to this loose living, allowing alcohol to be distilled for the troops and eventually decreeing:

> Throughout Egypt the use of a beverage prepared by some Moslems from hemp (hashish) as well as the smoking of the seeds of hemp, is prohibited. Habitual smokers and drinkers of this plant lose their reason and suffer from violent delirium in which they are liable to commit excesses of all kinds. . . . The preparation of hashish as a beverage is prohibited throughout Egypt. The doors of those cafes

and restaurants where it is supplied are to be walled up, and their proprietors imprisoned for three months.

It didn't work. The Egyptian population simply ignored the invaders' decrees. Moreover, the French soldiers returned home in defeat in 1801 not merely with a liking for cannabis, but with their own supplies of the drug. Scientific interest had been sparked too. Accompanying Napoleon's army on their Egyptian mission were 151 members of the Commission of the Sciences and Arts. From these scientists, the drug also made its way across the Mediterranean Sea. Until then, as Leslie Iversen has observed: 'Although cannabis had been cultivated in Europe for many centuries as a source of rope, canvas, and other cloths and in making paper, its inebriating effects were largely unknown.' In France at least, the cat was now out of the bag.

But usage was largely confined to an elite Parisian circle of writers, artists and bohemians. Among these were figures such as Balzac, Baudelaire, Dumas, Delacroix and Flaubert, who met in the secret Club des Hashischins, founded in 1844. The poet Théophile Gautier published an account of his first visit, 'obeying a mysterious summons, drafted in enigmatic terms understood by affiliates but unintelligible for others'. In a grand house on the Ile St Louis, an elaborate meal was prefaced with a spoonful of greenish 'jam', served on a small Japanese saucer. It didn't take long for Gautier to feel the jam's bite: 'The water I drank seemed the most exquisite wine, the meat, once in my mouth, became strawberries, the strawberries, meat. I could not have distinguished a fish from a cutlet.' As the minutes and hours passed, Gautier was transported. He basked in:

An undefinable sense of well-being, a calm without end. I was in the blessed phase of hashish which the Orientals call *kief*. No longer could I feel my body; the bonds between mind and matter were slender, I moved by simple desire into an environment which offered no resistance. . . . I understood at last the joys which, according to their degree of perfection, spirits and angels sense while floating across the ethers and heavens, and how eternity must pass in Paradise.

But this ecstatic tranquillity did not last. Eventually it was superseded by fear and paranoia. He heard a warning voice:

'Take care, for you are surrounded by enemies; invisible forces are trying to lure and hold you. You are a prisoner here: Try to escape and you shall see.' A veil was torn away from my mind's eye, and it became apparent to me that the club's members were none other than Cabalists and sorcerers who wished to sweep me to my doom. . . . I was overcome with despair, for, in lifting my hand to my skull, I found it open, and I lost consciousness.

For all the experiments of the Club des Haschischins, however, in the West cannabis was seldom consumed at scale until well into the twentieth century. Though the US Commissioner of the Federal Bureau of Narcotics, Harry J. Anslinger, would rail against 'reefer madness' in the 1930s, the drug was largely confined to Mexican immigrants in New Orleans and other southern cities and to the African-American jazz scene. Any possibility of a wider uptake was curtailed by the Marijuana Tax Act of 1937. In Europe, at least until the 1960s, hardly anyone was using the stuff – indeed it was so uncommon that the UK government did not feel the need to legislate until 1971.

What's your poison?

Things are, of course, very different now. Of all the controlled psychoactive substances, cannabis has become the world's favourite. Globally, around 180 million adults are estimated to use the drug. According to the 2022 edition of the Crime Survey for England and Wales, 16 per cent of people aged sixteen to twenty-four had taken cannabis at some point during the previous twelve months. Extending the age range to take in those under the age of sixty gives a prevalence rate of 7.4 per cent – around 2.5 million people. As in previous years, cannabis was by some margin the most consumed illegal drug in the UK. Cocaine, the second most prevalent, was used by 2 per cent of 16 to 59-year-olds. (This was a significant drop from previous years, probably due to the coronavirus lock-down: the partying paused.) In the US in 2021, 13 per cent of those aged twelve and above (36.4 million people) had used cannabis in the past month. The rate was highest among people aged eighteen to twenty-five, with almost a quarter (8.1 million) using cannabis in the previous month. Looking back over the past year, 52.5 million Americans over the age of twelve had taken cannabis.

Gauging whether cannabis use is increasing is difficult: very few countries have gathered this kind of historical data. But we do have statistics for the US, and they show a dramatic escalation in recent years – albeit with a Covid-related fall in the last couple of years. In fact, between 2002 and 2013 cannabis use in the country doubled. (Many US states have legalised medical use, and either decriminalised or legalised recreational use. But these initiatives largely date from after 2013.) In the UK, the number of young people using the drug has risen by 5 per cent since 2013. Between 1970 and 2002, the number of under-eighteens using cannabis is estimated to have grown eighteen-fold.

But though the consumption of cannabis in the West has escalated dramatically since Napoleonic times, public discourse hasn't changed as much as one might expect. Depending on where you stand, cannabis remains a dangerous substance that ought to be prohibited or a largely benign source of pleasure, relaxation and wellbeing. Cannabis is increasingly regarded as beneficial for a range of physical problems, and medical use has been legalised in several countries. But there is also much concern about its effects on mental health, and particularly its connection to psychosis.

Fuelling this concern is the fact that the cannabis routinely consumed today in Europe and the US is a turbocharged version of the relatively mild narcotic of the 1960s and 70s. Its potency has skyrocketed. What gives cannabis its kick is principally a chemical compound called delta-9-tetrahydrocannabinol, otherwise known as THC. Back in 1980 a typical US joint contained less than 2 per cent THC. By 2015, THC content had soared to as much as 20 per cent. It is much the same in the UK. The market is now dominated by sinsemilla or 'skunk' with an average THC content of 14 per cent. As the proportion of THC has grown, the amount of another important chemical has shrunk. Cannabidiol (CBD) doesn't possess psychoactive qualities; in fact, it counteracts the effects of THC. The cannabis resin that was once so widespread in Europe and the US was low in THC and relatively high in CBD. There is virtually no CBD in today's skunk.

So, what role does cannabis play in mental health problems? We know that cannabis can produce transitory psychotic experiences like Théophile Gautier's paranoia. But might there be long-lasting effects? Is it coincidental that some of my patients have used cannabis – and often continue to do so? Is cannabis a means of self-medication? Could it play a part in causing paranoia? Or is some other factor responsible for both paranoia and cannabis use?

It's worth noting, incidentally, that psychosis patients – like the rest of the UK population – are more likely to drink alcohol than they are to use cannabis. I see lots of people who drink in order to defuse their anxiety. And the evidence suggests alcohol – and drug – problems are more common among people with severe mental health problems. Unfortunately, alcohol tends to make things worse. Gradually, people end up needing more in order to relax. That interferes with their sleep, which as we saw in Chapter 7 only leads to more depression, anxiety and paranoia. We don't know enough yet about the links between alcohol and paranoia. But our analysis of the 2007 UK Adult Psychiatric Morbidity Survey certainly shows an association between alcohol dependence and paranoia. Moreover, the 2000 survey suggests that people with problematic drinking were more likely to report paranoid thoughts at the follow-up eighteen months later. Clearly, there's something going on here. What we need now is the research to determine precisely what that something is.

When it comes to cannabis and psychotic experiences like paranoia, we have numerous studies suggesting a link. Again, the question is: what is the nature of that connection? When, for example, Michael Wainberg and colleagues analysed data on 109,308 UK adults they discovered that cannabis users were significantly more likely to report psychotic experiences, especially paranoia. And the more cannabis they consumed, the more frequent and troubling their paranoia (this is what is known in the trade as a dose–response relationship). Our study of 1,714 members of the general population found that paranoia was much more common in the 38 per cent who'd used cannabis than in the others. Indeed, individuals with a history of cannabis use had almost twice the odds of reporting paranoid thoughts in the past month compared with individuals who had never taken cannabis.

These cross-sectional analyses are backed up by longitudinal studies that follow people over time. The first of these focused on fifty thousand young men – almost all aged between eighteen and twenty – conscripted into the Swedish military in 1969–70. (Service was compulsory for males in Sweden back then. Indeed, after a brief hiatus between 2010 and 2017 it is mandatory for both sexes today, though the numbers actually enlisted are far smaller now.) As part of the induction process, the recruits had been questioned about their substance use. Which drugs did they consume most often? How frequently did they use? What drug had they tried first? Fifteen years later the men who had smoked cannabis before joining the military were twice as likely to have subsequently developed schizophrenia. Similarly, in 2002 Jim van Os and colleagues assessed 4,045 members of the general population in the Netherlands and found that those who used cannabis were three times more likely to report paranoia and other psychotic experiences at follow-up assessments one and three years later. Again, the heavier the cannabis use, the more severe the paranoia.

Blotto in Oxford

It is clear then that cannabis use predicts later psychological problems, including paranoia. But can we go further? Can we prove that it is cannabis that contributes to the *cause* of those problems and, if so, how does it do it? In the very first experiment I undertook upon arrival in the Department of Psychiatry at Oxford, I endeavoured to find out. The study was the largest ever randomised controlled study of the effects of THC. We recruited 121 volunteers, all of whom had taken cannabis at least once before, and all of whom reported having experienced paranoid thoughts in the previous month (which is typical of half the population). None had ever been diagnosed with a mental health disorder.

It took no end of hassle to do it, but courtesy of my colleagues in pharmacology, we finally managed to secure vials of THC, imported from Switzerland. (There isn't much demand for injectable cannabis.) The volunteers were randomly chosen to receive an intravenous 1.5mg dose of either THC, the equivalent of a strong joint, or a saline placebo. It takes just five minutes for the THC to kick in, and the effects last around ninety minutes – which makes for a neat experimental window. So we carried out a slew of assessments before each participant had their injection and repeated those assessments while the THC was in their bloodstream.

As we've noted already in this book, it can be tricky to measure paranoia. Real threats do exist. When someone says they have been targeted, perhaps they are right. To combat that difficulty, we used a broad array of tests. The more we test, and the more varied the tests, the better our picture of what's going on. First up was a behavioural task: a short walk through the hospital with a stop at the canteen to buy a drink. The point here was for the participant to encounter other people – and, especially important, people they didn't know. We measured the participants' reactions by asking them immediately to complete a paranoia questionnaire. When that was done, it was time for a five-minute trip on our virtual London Underground train. Finally, we sat down with the participant to chat through their experiences, grading their responses on a further set of paranoia questionnaires.

Once all the many assessments were completed, the participant was invited – Oscar-style – to open an envelope. Inside was a piece of paper explaining which experimental group they had been part of. This was a big reveal for participants and researchers alike. No one, aside from the psychiatrists who had administered the injections, knew who had been dosed with cannabis and who had been given salty water. Sometimes everyone was surprised. I remember one guy who worked as a roadie in the music business. It was presumably his rock and roll lifestyle that explained why he was convinced he had been given the placebo. The THC left him cold. On the other hand, there were some in the control group who became extremely disinhibited: giggling and joking, flirting with the research team, and generally behaving like it was party time at the university. Except, of course, that for them it wasn't. And when they finally opened the fateful envelope, they sobered up with comic speed. The trip that hadn't been a trip was suddenly and definitively over. There is a priceless scene in Laurel and Hardy's 1930 movie *Blotto*, in which the boys smuggle a bottle of booze into a Prohibition-era nightclub, get uproariously drunk – and are then instantly jolted into chilly sobriety when Mrs Laurel reveals that what they have been drinking is, in fact, cold tea. It was rather like that, with the Warneford Hospital standing in for Stan and Ollie's Rainbow Club.

So, what did we observe in those who *had* been given THC? Well, it certainly made them more paranoid. Half of those in the THC group experienced paranoia, compared with 30 per cent of the placebo group. In other words, one in five had an increase in paranoia that was directly attributable to the THC. What this shows is that in people vulnerable to paranoia, cannabis can be a contributory cause. The drug produced other unsettling psychological effects, such as anxiety, worry, lowered mood and negative thoughts about the self. Short-term memory was impaired. (The musician Willie Nelson sees this as a benefit of cannabis: 'Otherwise you start remembering a lot of negative things that you're not supposed to remember. And the next

thing you know, you're back drinking whiskey.') And the THC
sparked a range of what psychologists call 'anomalous experiences': sounds seemed louder than usual and colours brighter;
thoughts appeared to echo in the individuals' minds; and time
seemed to be distorted. (Incidentally, we spoke to all the participants the next day to check that their paranoia had receded.
Happily, it had.)

Why is cannabis such a potent trigger for paranoia? Our
statistical analysis showed that the culprits in our experiment
were THC's negative effects on the individual's mood and view
of the self, and the anomalous sensory experiences it can
produce. (Short-term memory problems did not increase the
paranoia.) Negative emotions leave us feeling down and vulnerable. Worry leads us to the worst conclusions. So, when we try
to make sense of the anomalous experiences – when we try to
understand what's happening to us – the world can appear a
weird, frightening and hostile place. Hence the paranoia. Odd
experiences foster unusual thoughts. (Cannabis, of course, isn't
the only drug that can cause anomalous experiences. In the case
of hallucinogens like LSD, magic mushrooms and mescaline,
such experiences are precisely the attraction. I seldom see
patients who've been using these substances, but paranoia is
certainly a common feature of many bad trips.)

Whys and wherefores

Of course, although cannabis can cause long-lasting and sometimes severe paranoia, it doesn't do so for most people who
consume the drug (as we saw in our THC experiment). Take
the Swedish study we heard about earlier. Yes, heavy cannabis
users were much more likely to later receive a diagnosis of
schizophrenia. But even in that group only 3 per cent were

affected. What makes the difference? Our experiment suggested that, at the psychological level, paranoia is made more likely by negative emotions and the way we interpret anomalous experiences. But scientists have identified other factors too. One is the age at which someone starts consuming cannabis. The younger a person is when they begin regularly using the drug, the higher the probability of problems. That may be because the adolescent brain is still developing: its plasticity leaves it especially vulnerable to the effects of cannabis on various neurotransmitter systems. It's concerning then that more and more young people are using cannabis. Indeed, it's thought that around 40 per cent of today's fifteen-year-olds have tried it.

The potency of the drug also makes a difference to outcomes – and, as we have seen, the cannabis today's adolescents are consuming is often considerably stronger than in years gone by. This was demonstrated in a study led by Clare Mackie of the National Addiction Centre at the Institute of Psychiatry. Mackie recruited 467 sixteen- and seventeen-year-olds from schools and colleges across Greater London. Around 30 per cent of the group reported using cannabis in the previous twelve months. One in five of those users consumed skunk only (as opposed to milder herbal cannabis). And it was those guys – and two-thirds of them were male – who tended to experience paranoid thoughts. In fact, compared to non-users, skunk consumers were twice as likely to report paranoia.

Genes probably play a part too, though here the evidence is a little patchy. Michael Wainberg's study of 109,308 UK adults found that people with a genetic vulnerability to schizophrenia were much more susceptible to persecutory delusions (and other psychotic experiences such as hearing voices) after using cannabis. On the other hand, in a twin study of 4,830 sixteen-year-old pairs, Sania Shakoor and colleagues argued that though cannabis and psychotic experiences are strongly linked, genes

aren't especially significant. What matters more is likely to be
environmental factors. Here the finger has been pointed at
bullying, socioeconomic disadvantage and trauma. That's to
say, the people most at risk from cannabis-induced paranoia
– and other psychological problems – are those who've already
undergone material and emotional hardship. This seems plausible: we saw in Chapter 5 how potent trauma and bullying, for
example, can be in triggering paranoia. And indeed, an analysis
of 2,630 Australian cannabis users, aged sixteen to twenty-five,
found that those who had experienced childhood trauma were
more likely to report paranoia both when taking the drug and
afterwards too.

So where does this leave us in the debate regarding cannabis
and mental health? Well, it's clear that not everyone is at equal
risk of difficulties. The likelihood of things turning out badly is
dependent on a few key risk factors: the age of the individual;
the frequency with which they consume cannabis; the drug's
strength; and a likely mix of genetic, psychological and environmental influences. But for a small minority of people cannabis
can undoubtedly help trigger – and maintain – persecutory delusions. In fascinating work by Vicki Charles and Tim Weaver we
get to hear first-hand about the relationship between cannabis
and psychosis from fourteen patients in inner London. The
patients (almost all male) were aged between twenty-seven and
fifty-five. Most had used a variety of drugs – and almost everyone
still did. But all had started on cannabis while they were teenagers,
principally because it was what everyone else in their social circle
was doing. With one exception, the group had been using cannabis
for some time before they developed psychosis. Five of the fourteen believed their drug use had helped cause their mental health
problems, and five others thought it had made those difficulties
worse. This was doubtless why most had periodically stopped
using drugs: 'I think smoking [cannabis] helps sometimes, I think

it's a good way to let off steam but [pause] it's not good when you are having bad thoughts all the time.' But the perceived advantages always drew people back: 'It [cannabis] just relaxed me. . . . I can be angry. If I smoke a spliff I would just relax, I will just chill. I won't be bothered . . . but if I do any "A" class, cocaine or crack or ecstasy, then that's different. It just sends me Jekyll and Hyde.' For some, cannabis was seen as a vital means to counteract the negative side effects of antipsychotic drugs. Cannabis had become their 'medicine'.

A team at the University of Sheffield led by Helen Childs spoke to seven young adults being treated for psychosis. All said they'd used cannabis regularly in the past and/or were currently doing so. Like the people Charles and Weaver spoke to, the Sheffield cohort had started young: anywhere from eleven to fourteen. None of them recalled having experienced any mental health issues by this point. Again, as with the London group social factors had been decisive in prompting this early experimentation: 'everyone smoked it at school'; 'the cooler kids did it and, well, it was kind of like, there was always that kind of chicness about it'. These times were remembered fondly: 'For the first few years I was smoking it . . . it just either made me laugh or made me like "hello" and really, really stoned but it never gave me any psychosis.' Gradually though they'd all upped their intake, in some cases to the point where they felt physically addicted: 'all day every day, when I got up I'd light a spliff'. By that stage, cannabis was becoming much less fun: 'I started getting really freaked out and thinking all my friends were evil and like, I worked out how they had all these plots against me.' Looking back, everyone noted a connection between their cannabis use and feelings of paranoia and other distressing experiences, though they sometimes hadn't been able to make sense of it at the time:

'. . . it sort of triggers like outlandish thoughts and concepts . . . I remember before, er, thinking . . . other people could actually hear what was going on in my head and interact with it and stuff like that . . . but because you're under the influence of cannabis it's, it makes it easier to believe these sort of f-fantasy ideas.'

'. . . it would feel like, say the TV was on and the TV was, would get like slightly louder and the room would go slightly more orange and you'd get like a spotlight almost coming onto you.'

For some of the participants, enough was enough: 'if I smoked it, I know it would just send me like absolutely scared shitless I think.' Others continued but modified their usage according to the state of their mental health, cutting back when 'a murmur' was detected. And for one person, cannabis was seen as a (temporary) remedy for paranoia: 'all my thoughts are just pushed away and . . . I feel good for a bit but once . . . it's gone, it, it just, it just goes back to normal if not worser.'

Nicotine

'What has happened to individual freedom and our respect for the human dignity of New York City's most vulnerable citizens – the seriously and chronically mentally ill? Why does Bellevue Hospital force patients to go cold turkey? Please create a discrete smoking area for all your psychiatric patients.'

National Alliance for the Mentally Ill and Friends and Advocates of the Mentally Ill campaign literature (1990)

When I first started working at the Institute of Psychiatry, the waiting room was permeated by cigarette smoke. This wasn't surprising: it seemed like almost every patient I saw was a smoker. Even today, rates are around three times higher in people diagnosed with schizophrenia, with more than 60 per cent smoking. And those 60 per cent smoke more heavily than other people. Why?

The conventional view has been that smoking is an attempt to cope with mental health problems – a kind of self-medication. One certainly hears this from patients: 'Smoking is quite relaxing, and goes well with alcohol, it is a way to give yourself a break'; 'Cigarettes would calm me down, I'd experience stress and think: "I need a fag", it was a way of coping with stress.'

Interestingly, however, documents released in the late 1990s revealed that a vigorous proponent of this idea had been the tobacco industry. These companies had funded research designed to demonstrate the benefits of smoking for people with serious mental health difficulties, had supplied cigarettes to psychiatric institutions (sometimes free and sometimes in response to begging letters from clinicians), and had frustrated efforts to ban smoking in hospitals. A 1986 Philip Morris advertisement perhaps says all that needs to be said on the matter:

Schizophrenic: Big taste, lower tar, all in one. For New Merit, having two sides is just normal behaviour.

It also seems to me that many patients have a lot of time on their hands and smoking is one way of filling it. Smoking can help facilitate social contact too – a big plus for people whose mental health problems can often leave them feeling isolated. Now, however, researchers are exploring a couple of very different perspectives on the phenomenon. First is the idea that nicotine may actually be a contributory cause of paranoia and other psychotic experiences, right up to and including schizo-phrenia. The second is that smoking and schizophrenia share a genetic component: the genes that make a person more likely to become dependent on nicotine also increase the chance of that individual developing psychosis.

There is certainly evidence that adults who smoke tobacco regularly are more likely to go on to experience paranoia: it increases the odds by anywhere between 20 and 47 per cent. And those who begin smoking during adolescence are especially vulnerable. The study by Clare Mackie we looked at earlier in this chapter focused on skunk use. But it also found a link between paranoia and nicotine, even for adolescents who used e-cigarettes. This is concerning given that e-cigarette use seems to be on the rise among young people in the US and in those European countries for which historical data is available.

And the genetic dimension? In a study led by Wikus Barkhuizen and Angelica Ronald at the University of London's Centre for Brain and Cognitive Development, we analysed data on 3,878 sixteen-year-old twins. The association between smoking and paranoia was modest. Nevertheless, the 5 per cent who described themselves as regular smokers (defined as having consumed fifty or more cigarettes during their lifetime) were also those most likely to report paranoia and other psychotic experiences. Again, we saw a dose–response relationship, with occasional smokers scoring higher than non-smokers for paranoia and, in turn, regular smokers outscoring occasional smokers. That smoking and paranoia often occur in the same people doesn't, of course, mean that there is a causal connection. And yet we found a big genetic crossover between smoking and paranoia. In fact, almost all the association between the two could be explained by shared genetic factors. In other words, the reason people smoke and become paranoid is, genetically at least, the same. (DNA may not always exert its influence directly. In a gene–environment interaction, the genes involved in paranoia can lead us into life situations that make tobacco use more likely, and vice versa.)

I should caution that research on the links between smoking and paranoia is at an early stage. We don't know, for example, whether the genetic theory stands up. If it's true that smoking can be a cause of paranoia, we don't know how exactly it does so. What are the psychological mechanisms at play? In fact, it isn't just paranoia and smoking that merits more attention. Smoking is associated with a broad spectrum of psychological problems, including the most common conditions. Thirty-seven per cent of people with depression smoke, for example. Doubtless the psychological ramifications of smoking have been overshadowed by its catastrophic physical toxicity. Nevertheless, given that 1.3 billion people in the world are smokers, the fact that we understand relatively little about the interaction between tobacco and mental health problems seems a big oversight.

'The pharmakon [drug],' wrote Jacques Derrida, 'will always be understood both as antidote and as poison.' Most people use cannabis without adverse effects, and indeed with plenty of pleasant ones. (At a stretch, one could say something similar about tobacco.) And yet the 'antidote' can also function as a poison. Cannabis can trigger paranoia – both short-term and, in some cases, severe enough to require clinical intervention. With millions of people around the world consuming unprecedentedly potent cannabis, and doing so at an increasingly young age, this is a public health issue that isn't about to disappear any time soon.

10.

The voices in my head

'I used to find it really, really difficult to go out because the fear was so strong. I'd be very frightened just to walk down the road. I was fearful that somebody would pass me in a car, get out and attack me. Because everything was so frightening, I would isolate myself. I wouldn't actually go out very often.

I can remember being very frightened of people looking at me. When we're out and about, we look at each other. We people-watch. But I would interpret a look as meaning that somebody would want to hurt me. The voices would feed into that – they were persecutory voices. I thought everyone could read my mind as well, so that was quite frightening. I didn't like to be around other people. The voices would tell me they were psychic so I would walk around with my head down looking at the floor. I didn't want to see anything that was going on around me because it could possibly trigger something.'

'Why did you think people might be picking on you?'

'I don't know. I remember being bullied quite badly at work when I first left home. It wasn't very pleasant, and it ended up that I would just not go to work. And then I think over time those kinds of thoughts would just snowball. I would even be paranoid about my closest friends. And at school as well. I

didn't fare particularly well at school. I think for quite a lot of my life I've looked at the world as quite a scary place.

I was worried that my house was being bugged and there were cameras in my house. I know they can make very, very small cameras these days. So, I thought if I looked, I'd never find it. I remember when I used to have really, really bad voices I thought I'd put on some music and that would distract me from the voices. But they would come out of the stereo speakers or the television.

I remember I had a little radio at one point, and I was really worried that there was some kind of bug in the radio. I remember taking it apart and really looking to see if I could find anything in there. And there wasn't. I thought mobile phones were another way that people were tracking what I was doing.'

'What sort of information do you think they were trying to track?'

'Stuff that maybe they could use against me. There was a link between being monitored and the voices. I thought that they were gathering information that they could then use to taunt me. A lot of it would just go round and round and round in my head. It was exhausting. Absolutely exhausting.'

Understanding voice hearing

'Hearing voices no one else can hear isn't a good sign, even in the wizarding world.'

J. K. Rowling, *Harry Potter and the Chamber of Secrets* (1998)

Today we are used to public figures talking candidly about their depression or anxiety. It's a welcome change from the silence that used to surround mental health problems. Yet some experiences remain taboo. Hearing voices, described so well by Toby in the account that opens this chapter, is one of them. What do we mean by hearing voices? We're dealing here with a form of hallucination. It's an experience that occurs without an appropriate stimulus (you hear a voice, but no one is speaking). It has the same effect as it would if the voice were real. And it isn't consciously controlled by the person experiencing the hallucination.

Sometimes the voices seem to be located in the hearer's head. More often it feels as though they come from outside – from someone in the same room, for instance. The mechanism isn't well understood. But at a psychological level we can think of it as a misattribution of internal processes to external stimuli. Our brain mistakes inner speech, or memories, for the voice of another person. Brain scans bear this out. When an individual experiences an auditory hallucination, blood flows to Broca's area, a part of the brain heavily involved in language production. Other studies have found a surge of activity in areas of the brain that process external sounds and those involved in verbal memory. Of course, the key question is why this happens for some people and not others. To date, however, that's a question without an answer. There are many theories, but no hard evidence. Similarly, we don't know why some people hear one voice while others hear multiple voices. We don't know why some people hear voices occasionally and others repeatedly. And we don't know why some people's voices are hostile while the voices heard by others are friendly. Certain experiences seem to crop up frequently among voice hearers, and especially those whose voices are nasty: for example, sleep problems, anxiety, stress, isolation and trauma. But of course, many people have these experiences without hearing voices.

Although we don't tend to talk about it, hallucinations are

much more common than we might assume. Like paranoia, there is a spectrum. A relatively small number of people struggle with persistent upsetting hallucinations – and those are the people I see in clinic. But lots more experience sporadic hallucinations. All in all, around 4 per cent of the general population – excluding those with psychosis – report that, in the previous twelve months, they have heard or seen things that others couldn't. Around 0.7 per cent have heard voices when there was no one around to account for it. It isn't always an unpleasant experience. Some people welcome their voices, which can be a source of support and advice, spiritual guidance, even creativity. Moreover, though hearing voices is generally regarded as a frightening sign of mental health problems in the West, attitudes can vary hugely across societies. Shamanic cultures, for example, understand hearing voices as communication from the spirits. And when the American anthropologist Tanya Luhrmann interviewed patients diagnosed with schizophrenia in San Mateo in California, Chennai in India, and Accra in Ghana, she found:

> Striking differences in the quality of the voice-hearing experience, and particularly in the quality of relationship with the speaker of the voice. Many participants in the Chennai and Accra samples insisted that their predominant or even only experience of the voices was positive . . . Not one American did so. Many in the Chennai and Accra samples seemed to experience their voices as people: the voice was that of a human the participant knew, such as a brother or a neighbour, or a human-like spirit whom the participant also knew. These respondents seemed to have real human relationships with the voices – sometimes even when they did not like them. This was less typical of the San Mateo sample, whose reported experiences were markedly more violent, harsher and more hated.

Certain life events are more likely to trigger hallucinations. It is not uncommon, for instance, for the bereaved to hear the voice of their loved one. In one study of fifty people who had lost a spouse, a third reported seeing, hearing and talking to their deceased partner. Some people experience hallucinations as they pass from sleep to wakefulness, and vice versa. (These are known as hypnopompic and hypnagogic hallucinations, respectively.) A survey of nearly five thousand people in the UK found that 37 per cent reported hypnagogic hallucinations while they were falling asleep, and 12.5 per cent reported hypnopompic ones as they were waking up. Those in the sample with insomnia, excessive daytime sleepiness or mental health problems were more susceptible.

Going without sufficient sleep is likely to produce hallucinations. Rémy Hurdiel and colleagues analysed the experience of sailors in a single-handed transatlantic race. The first leg lasted six to eight days and took the competitors from La Rochelle in France to the island of Madeira, which lies around three hundred miles west of Morocco. The second leg was even more demanding, taking the boats over three thousand nautical miles from Madeira to Salvador de Bahia in Brazil – a trip that for some lasted more than three weeks. Solo sailing naturally requires more or less constant alertness. The sailors estimated that they managed around four to five hours of sleep in every twenty-four hours, often comprising two or three hours at night and a nap in the afternoon. It was no surprise that this chronic sleep deprivation resulted in the sailors making errors, undergoing mood swings – and experiencing both visual and auditory hallucinations.

Also no surprise is the observation that drugs can cause us to perceive things that don't have a basis in the external world. Indeed, it's precisely the power to alter perception that gives recreational drugs much of their appeal. ('I see better days and

I do better things,' as Bob Dylan put it.) There is certainly a link between drug taking and hearing hostile voices. But it is not just recreational drugs that can trigger hallucinations. In the last few years, it has become evident that the heavy medication used in operations and intensive care can cause profound perceptual disturbance. Intensive care units can bring additional complicating factors. Patients may be sleep deprived and disorientated. Infection can cause delirium. The result can be nightmarish hallucinations:

> 'There were puffin birds jumping out of the curtains with toy guns, firing blood at me. I kept wiping my face . . . There were loads of birds jumping on the next bed . . . laughing at each other. Completely crazy. I was really scared. I didn't say anything to anyone.'

> 'Before I knew it, a nurse came upon me. She gave me the injection. There were people there with cloaks like an abbot, I couldn't see their faces. They were . . . families who would take your soul . . . They would envelop you . . . suck you up and move on . . . I jumped out and got away but ended up in a coffin in a chapel of rest.'

Voices and paranoia

If hearing voices is still beyond the pale, so too, I would argue, are paranoid delusions. In fact, the two often occur together. In this respect Toby, who we heard from at the beginning of this chapter, is typical of the patients I see with persecutory delusions, about half of whom also experience auditory hallucinations. As Toby found, the voices seed, and cultivate, paranoia. This works in two ways. First, the voices encourage a sense of vulnerability. As we have seen repeatedly in this book, paranoia feeds on that vulnerability: 'telling me things like I'm worthless and you know, you don't deserve to be here'; 'everybody else hates you and they don't need you and they think the worst of you. And um, just that you are you know just a complete disappointment.'

The voices probe anxieties, seek out insecurities. They find a tender spot and home in on it, again and again. For many of us, the way we look is just such a spot. That is certainly true for people with persecutory delusions, as we saw in Chapter 8. And if they hear voices, it is a worry that those voices are likely to seize upon: 'You are ugly. You don't deserve nobody. You're ugly, people are looking at you, look at them looking at you.'

When Felicity Waite in my team interviewed sixty patients (comprising slightly more men than women) who reported hearing voices at least once a week, she discovered that 90 per cent endured regular negative remarks about their appearance: telling them that they were, for example, fat or ugly. For 50 per cent, those comments occurred every single day.

The second way in which voices fuel paranoia is more direct. They explicitly tell the person about a threat. Sometimes the voice figures as the putative perpetrator. Sometimes other people are the source of danger: 'The voices had me believing that I wouldn't be waking up in the morning. And um they said they were going to skin me um, rape me, all this horrible stuff'; 'They encouraged me to think that my mother and her husband and some of my friends were all, all kind of serial killers'; 'They were on about my neighbour that lives upstairs and they said they were going to hurt the kids and so I ran up the stairs.'

Imagine having to listen to comments like this, over and over again, day after day. Small wonder then that people who hear these kinds of voices are much more likely to experience depression, anxiety and suicidal thoughts – as well as severe paranoia:

'it's a scary, scary, scary, scary situation, I've had more fear in the last two years than anywhere in my life'; 'The worst thing is to feel that self-destructive sort of "oh, I've got a solution for all this, I will just end it."'

'What have I done?'

We know that the level of distress caused by voices depends on the hearer's interpretation of those voices. Just like any other experience, our response is determined by how we construe the meaning. Clearly, it is not easy to shrug off being told that you are worthless, that you are weak, that just by stepping outside the front door you are putting yourself in danger. But people can learn to manage their voices. They can reduce the distress those voices cause. And as clinicians, we're in a much better position to help if we understand why patients frequently listen to and believe hostile voices, even when they know the voices are trying to get at them. Bryony Sheaves from my team has delivered new insights into this key question. In the first stage of her research Bryony spoke to fifteen people being treated in NHS services for psychosis. All heard hostile voices every day and had done so for at least the previous three months. From those conversations six major themes emerged – six types of reasons why the participants listened to, and believed, their voices.

First was a desire to understand the voices. Who is speaking? And why? 'I will look around, I will try and work out who is saying it, why they are saying it, I don't understand, what have I done?' Making sense of what was happening was hard: 'I didn't really know that much about hearing voices, so I sort of just believed it.'

For some of the people Bryony interviewed, the voices provided essential information about possible threats: 'I've got to listen to this because I need to know what they are planning to do to me so I can be prepared.' To avert harm, people sometimes tried to negotiate with their voices: 'I would like bargain with them, like if I do it more or if I do it better will you make sure something bad doesn't happen to me?' Most of the interviewees had tried confronting the voices: 'I was just taking them on, I was like I'm not having this any more . . . you are not going to rule over me all the time.' But there was a fear that ignoring the voices would lead to harm: 'Oh, they will screw me more.'

'I didn't know I was ill. I thought that was the way it was.' This natural tendency to accept what our senses tell us was the third reason why Bryony's interviewees engaged with their voices. After all, why would you question something that seems so real? And if the voices threatened to kill you, was that really so unlikely? For one individual, pondering the events of the Second World War provided ample evidence for the truth of what the voices were saying: 'And you think well, those people were totally evil, they would be thinking the same kind of things in terms of murdering anything they didn't like.' Other types of hallucination seem to substantiate the voices: 'they were telling me that like a woman was coming with a gun . . . she would find a way to shoot me . . . I laid on my bed like battling about it and then I looked up and like in the doorway . . . she was just stood there.'

It can be difficult to resist the voices when they sound like someone you know: 'I think I find it harder to rationalise than say if it was a stranger in a café because I don't know their voice from Adam.' It's especially tricky if the voice appears to belong to someone you are close to, if it's 'one of the voices that you trust more than anything'. And the voice may not simply sound familiar. The words spoken can seem eerily plausible too: 'they are doing exactly what they did when I fell out with them . . . I think they are just trying to finish the job.' For a minority, the voices they hear are a direct memory of past experiences and often abuse – a horrible flashback that is reminiscent of post-traumatic stress disorder.

However much the interviewees sought to dismiss them, they were usually bested by the persistence, cunning, and sometimes downright aggression of the voices. 'I think to myself why are you listening, it's not worth listening to. But obviously that's easier said than done if you . . . had constant noise and voices for like two, three, four, five days.' For some interviewees it was when the voices shrank to a whisper that they captured their hearers' attention: 'it makes you want to listen, the voices, the voices do it as well and it just makes you want to listen to them.' For others, the voices were so loud and confrontational that they were impossible to ignore. And it wasn't only their volume or tone that made them compelling. Several people talked about the voices deliberately trying to intrigue them: 'the memories like, when they say things from the past and that, things you had forgotten like and you remember it. Sort of grabs your attention.'

Lastly, the interviewees described being ground down by the voices. 'Every day I was trying to battle the thing I couldn't win.' Having been constantly got at, threatened and belittled, they had exhausted the reserves of emotional energy required to combat the voices. And the voices seemed to know exactly when to take advantage: 'it's like guerrilla warfare . . . they are waiting until I'm down and out and vulnerable, weak, and then they will attack.' When that vulnerability stems in part from pre-existing problems, the voices have another base on which to build: 'I mean I suffer from depression . . . you have always got that thing in the back of your mind that you are . . . no good, a no-good character.'

Sleeping badly doesn't help: 'when I haven't slept that's, that's when I struggle to, to even like er, I struggle to like even make them stop'. As we saw in Chapter 7, sleep problems are prevalent – indeed, they are the norm – in people diagnosed with psychosis. Inactivity and isolation also left the interviewees more vulnerable to their voices. Again, this is not an uncommon problem for people with psychosis, two-thirds of whom experience clinical levels of agoraphobia. In some cases, people become more or less housebound, so intense is their fear of what might happen were they to leave the home. 'It becomes monotonous. Your brain is going to look for something of interest at some point, it's going to start inventing things because you get up, you watch TV, you go to the toilet, you watch TV, you go to bed, you don't do anything. Do that for five years you will lose your mind.'

Isolation

'. . . *the worst thing I did was when I was sixteen I didn't tell anyone. And then I ended up like having a complete breakdown when I was eighteen and I think that could have been averted if I had actually reached out to someone.*'

Overcoming isolation to form positive relationships with other people is a huge factor in recovery from psychosis. But that means escaping from a nasty loop in which isolation strengthens the hold exerted by the voices, which in turn makes it more difficult for the individual to build those healing relationships. In a separate study involving the same fifteen participants, Bryony Sheaves set out to discover more about what it's like to be around other people when you're hearing hostile voices.

The short answer is that it can be extremely difficult, not least because the voices often seem hellbent on fostering mistrust: 'the voices are telling me people are going to hurt me . . . I can't really walk past people.' This paranoia can present challenges for clinicians as we endeavour to build trust and rapport with patients. One interviewee recalled how their voice warned them: 'just because you have had like one meeting . . . they would be like don't think . . . they are not going to do anything.'

There were other ways in which the voices made it hard to connect with other people. If they hadn't experienced it themselves, how could anyone truly appreciate what it's like to hear voices? 'It's difficult for anyone who hasn't been through it . . . to understand.' And that failure of understanding was sometimes combined with a perceived lack of empathy: 'They all say it's completely in my head and there's no reality attached to it whatsoever . . . no one really understands it.'

On the other hand, many of the group deliberately shielded their loved ones from the reality of the voices: 'I would rather it just scared me than scared anybody else.' They worried about the effect on relationships of talking openly about their experiences: 'imagine there are two pillars supporting the roof and I sort of broke down and he has to be even stronger.' In some cases, there was a worry that the voices might target friends and family members: 'if I told someone else they would also know, and then the [voices] would try and kill them as well.' There was another very powerful reason why the interviewees often preferred to keep the voices to themselves – they feared rejection: 'I haven't told anyone you know, even, even my best friend I would never tell them in this much detail . . . it's you know it sounds mad isn't it, which it is you know.' The voices sometimes stoked this anxiety: 'it's always been [the voices saying] that everybody else hates you and they don't need you and they think the worst of you.'

When you're hearing hostile voices, just carrying on a conversation with other people can rapidly become exhausting. Your attention is divided between the person you're with and the voices you hear, and it's not always easy to tell one from the other: 'sometimes like I hear my name um being called . . . but sometimes somebody is actually calling me and it's like am I thinking or hearing it?' Maintaining concentration can be draining: 'after ten minutes I was just so exhausted I said look I can't talk anymore.' Then there's the fear that the voices are listening to what you say: 'that's why I stop myself at certain points and I have to go no . . . I'm not going to talk about that.' Or that just being around other people will trigger the voices: '[the voices] can possess people around me and, and they can start talking through these people. And it's like they are talking at me directly.'

Given all this, it's not surprising that many people who hear hostile voices retreat into themselves: 'You know you withdraw, you don't want to talk to people'; 'The only people that I'm really in contact with on a kind of regular basis, is my mum and her husband. I don't really speak to him much, I speak to my mum occasionally.' The interviewees talked about being present physically but absent emotionally: 'I would go and see my family, but I wouldn't say anything to them really.' The voices may have profoundly affected the individual's wellbeing. But that didn't make it any easier to open up about what they were going through. One individual had been hearing hostile voices for fifteen years, and yet had never said a word about it to family and friends. It is a very heavy load to carry alone.

Pushed into isolation by the voices, the lack of social connection only exacerbated the problem: 'Not talking to people just made myself worse.' Partly this was because the voices often thrive on boredom: 'when I am kind of on my own . . . they kind of really do occupy my kind of attention.' If the hearer is alone, the voices seem more compelling and credible than ever: 'you could beat any of the strongest people down by you know making them solitary and then keep telling them something until they believed it.' Conversely, when people find a way to spend positive time with others the voices can become less intrusive: 'I'm focused on the person . . . without even thinking about it I'm just not hearing the voices as much.' Being candid about hearing voices helps: 'the more I could open up, the more I let my mates know, the more everything has settled down really.' The perspective of others can help loosen the voices' hold: '[the voices] are telling me a red van is going to . . . pull me in and drive me off . . . if I voice it and then my mate can be like it's just your voices babe, like look around there's no red van.'

'I don't need to feel ashamed': Voices and therapy

'I try to tell myself in my mind that nobody is watching me and that I'm just paranoid but then other voices from people I don't even know enter my mind and laugh and say things like "Yes, we are silly", "We're always watching you." Then they get louder and I can't really shut them up or fight them. They all sit with me when I'm using the bathroom watching me, or when I'm in my room. They make me laugh, they argue with me and make me mad, sometimes they make me cry.'

Hostile voices often play a big part in persecutory delusions. So tackling them is a clinical priority. But doing so is far from straightforward. Voices that have been continually intruding for months or even years on end are unlikely suddenly to disappear, no matter how much therapist and patient desire it. Instead, I work with the patient to reduce the frequency and power of the voices. Rather than simply accepting what the voices say, I want the patient to weigh up the evidence and decide for themselves. As one patient put it, what we are trying to build is the 'confidence to believe in my mind a little bit maybe, rather than the voices'.

To achieve this, it's important to create an environment in which the patient feels able to talk about their experiences. This may seem obvious; unless the patient is willing to communicate their thoughts and feelings, no therapy can succeed. Nonetheless, it can be especially significant in the case of people who are hearing voices, because they usually assume that this is an experience that is best kept to themselves. Empathy, as always, is vital. I can't lose sight of how distressing it can be to hear hostile voices. I want the person to share, and I want them to know that it's okay to do so. But it needs to happen at their own pace.

Then I'm keen to find out what triggers the voices. In what situations are they most likely to occur? I call these situations 'hot spots' and often they happen when the individual is bored or anxious. Poor sleep, alcohol or drugs, and stressful situations can be a contributory factor. If the voices are more or less continuous, it's a question of identifying the moments when they fall silent, however briefly – first thing in the morning, for instance, or when the person is humming or singing. These are the 'good spots', and my objective is to encourage more of them and fewer of the hot spots.

Lastly but most importantly, therapy is about changing the individual's relationship with what their voices say. What I'm after is to encourage the patient to venture a new perspective on their voices. To see things differently. To appreciate that what the voices tell them may not be accurate or helpful, and that other interpretations are possible. That process sometimes involves learning that these experiences are much more common than the patient might suppose. And that it is possible to live in relative harmony with the voices, to get to the place that a participant in Bryony Sheaves' study described: 'I've accepted that the voices are part of my life. I don't need to feel ashamed.' Talking to other voice hearers can be a big help: 'I can talk freely and not worry they'll judge me or get upset.' A few years back, that would have been difficult to organise. But things began to change when in 1987 Patsy Hage appeared on a Dutch TV talk show. Hage was then thirty-one years old. Having heard voices since she was eight, Hage seemed to have reached the end of the road. 'What I'm afraid of,' she told the show's host, 'is that this ends with a life where I'm just stuck sitting in a chair at home, not allowed to meet anyone or do anything, and that I end up climbing the walls with loneliness and isolation.' With Hage in the studio that evening was her psychiatrist, Marius Romme. Like his patient, Romme was at a loss: 'Helping her so that the voices go away is not something psychiatry can do.' What Hage and Romme wanted was advice from the show's audience. Was it possible to live productively with voices and, if so, how? They were astonished by the response to their appearance. Five hundred people contacted the programme to say that they heard voices. And a third of those said that they could indeed cope. Hage and Romme, together with the researcher Sandra Escher, invited many of those respondents to the first Hearing Voices Congress later that year. It was the start of the Hearing Voices Movement. Today there are groups across the world, with more than one hundred and eighty in the UK alone. Fundamental to the movement is the idea that hearing voices is a normal part of human experience and a meaningful response to life events – and that discussing them with other voice hearers can be an effective way of learning to cope.

To close this chapter, here is the psychologist Eleanor Longden, whose remarkable TED Talk 'The voices in my head' has been viewed online over six million times. Longden is carrying out her own research on how best to talk about voices in therapy.

She is an eloquent spokesperson for the Hearing Voices Movement, and a potent illustration of the fact that, despite the apparent hopelessness of one's situation, it is possible to make peace with one's voices:

By now I was so tormented by my voices that I'd attempted to drill a hole in my head in order to get them out . . . Many people have harmed me in my life, and I remember them all, but the memories grow pale and faint in comparison with the people who've helped me. . . . They helped me understand what I'd always suspected: that my voices were a meaningful response to painful life events, particularly childhood events, and as such were not my enemies but a source of insight into solvable emotional problems. . . . Not as an abstract symptom of illness to be endured but as a complex, meaningful, and significant experience to be explored. . . . I realised that the most hostile and aggressive voices actually represented the parts of me that had been hurt most profoundly, and as such it was these voices that needed to be shown the greatest compassion and care.

11.

How do I know this?

'Therefore you don't have a single answer to your questions?'
'Adso, if I did I would teach theology in Paris.'
'In Paris do they always have the true answer?'
'Never,' William said, 'but they are very sure of their errors.'
'And you,' I said with childish impertinence, 'never commit errors?'
'Often,' he answered. 'But instead of conceiving only one, I imagine many, so I become the slave of none.'
Umberto Eco, *The Name of the Rose* (1980)

In 1979 Robert Chapman was working as a machinist for a few months before attending college. He'd moved out of the family home and into the local YMCA. Things seemed to be going pretty well: 'I liked my job, the pay, and the people I worked for. And I was going to college in the fall. In addition, I worked week-ends at the Comedy Club doing standup.' Gradually, however, Chapman became convinced of two things. First, that he possessed unique insight into the world. And second, that his ideas were so remarkable that other people were stealing them. In time, he also came to believe that some of his thoughts were being forcefully inserted into his mind.

When Chapman began college, the situation deteriorated: 'I could not help but conclude that my mind was going to die from a telepathic thrashing – that my mind would be left in ruin to the point of total insanity, that I would literally lose my whole mind. I believed I was being persecuted, plotted against, by telepathic means.' His ambitions changed: rather than completing college he would become rich and successful by pursuing his 'new and inventive ideas'. But he was in the grip of a destructive paranoia: 'People were plotting against me, announcers on TV and radio were referring to me, people were planning to make me go crazy and subdue me. I felt that I didn't exist physically. I thought a celestial or psychic agent was after me. I received straight F's on my college progress report.'

In the spring of 1980 Chapman admitted himself to a psychiatric ward, received a diagnosis of schizophrenia, and began taking antipsychotic medication. Yet the next five years brought little improvement. Abandoning thoughts of gaining his college degree, he stayed up late working on his 'inventions':

> But no matter where I went, the tormenting thoughts would not cease. I felt powerless, horrified, and hindered now that my education was set aside. . . . every day I thought I was going to die from whoever was monitoring my thoughts and inserting unwanted thoughts into my mind. I felt so isolated, even when I was in a crowd. I thought that someone around me might be the one who was doing this to me, but I would never know who.

'The prognosis for Rob is not very good. . . . Rob is quite out of touch with reality. He has very poor insight. His present goals are totally unrealistic.' This was one clinician's summation of Chapman's condition in May 1982. As it turned out, from this very low ebb things slowly began to turn around. Chapman resolved to devise his own recovery plan: 'I reasoned that if some of my thoughts were disturbed, I could use my unaffected mind to think myself well again.' At the core of that plan was the insight that his delusions could be *doubted*. 'How is it that I have been feeling very paranoid about being persecuted for so long, yet I haven't been killed, assassinated, kidnapped, or imprisoned? For so long, I have suspected that a plot is being undertaken to victimise me, but nothing along these lines has taken place? I have not disappeared.' Doubt gave Chapman the springboard to interrogate the case for and against each of his delusions:

> I put on my detective cap. I would test out arguments. I tried to develop the strongest arguments possible against the falsehoods. I made a list of all the rational alternatives that I could think of. I looked for evidence for what really was happening and what really wasn't happening. I asked myself, 'How do I know this?' Did I actually see it or just a 'sign' of it? Did I really hear it, or could I have misinterpreted what I heard? Did I smell, taste, or feel it? Did someone tell me this? Is most of my evidence beyond my senses or interpretations of signs and symbols? . . . Since I realised I had a bias toward thinking meager evidence confirmed my false beliefs, I looked particularly hard for disconfirming evidence.

As the months rolled by, Chapman doggedly pursued his homemade therapy: 'It can take years to dismiss a belief altogether. Since I guess I had a tendency to jump to conclusions or make thinking errors, a delusion would sometimes resurface after I had thought I had worked on it enough. I investigated further, developing counterarguments at my scared, crawling pace.' One by one, and over a period of three years, Chapman overcame his delusions. As his condition improved, he was gradually able to stop taking antipsychotic medication. Eight years after dropping out of college, he returned to study graphic design. He wrote extensively about his mental health problems, and the techniques he had used for recovery. Today he works as a mental health adviser.

Jumping to conclusions

'You don't need proof when you have instinct.'
Reservoir Dogs (1992)

As we have observed already, patients' understanding of their experience often outstrips that of their clinicians. That was certainly true in Robert Chapman's case. Long before the mental health profession cottoned on, Chapman saw that his paranoia was rooted in, and enabled by, the way he reasoned – the patterns of thought he used when trying to make sense of the world. In stark contrast to his later strategy, Chapman had for years assumed that his delusional beliefs were accurate and important: 'The thoughts were so strong and seemed so unique, how could I ignore them?' As his paranoia grew, it increasingly dictated his view of the world: 'I often misinterpreted real-life occurrences such as the behaviors of others as somehow related to those conspiring against me. When people passed by (police cruisers, door-to-door salespeople), I thought they must be there to spy on me.' There was no scepticism, no doubt, no consideration of alternative interpretations: 'I thought I "knew." Knowing preceded thinking.'

As it happens, this rush to judgement is typical of people with delusions. In 2002 I asked one hundred psychosis patients two questions:

– Can you think of any other explanations for the experiences that you have described?

– Are there any other reasons – other than [the delusional belief] – that could possibly account for these experiences even if you think they are very unlikely?

In most cases these experiences were mundane, everyday events – an exchange of glances, a collision in the street, a jumble of litter near the patient's front door. Yet three-quarters of the group could think of no explanation other than their delusion. Not a single alternative. Nothing. This is pretty remarkable. After all, I wasn't asking for a more plausible interpretation of the event, just a different one. I see this all the time with patients in clinic. On the rare occasions when someone hazards an alternative explanation it is usually that they are ill. This was certainly the case in my survey. Of the 25 per cent who did suggest alternatives, almost all only suggested a single additional explanation – typically related to psychiatric illness. But this is a general interpretation for a particular event. It's a 'macro' rather than a 'micro' perspective. And from up there it's much harder to focus on the specifics of an event. Moreover, even those who ventured the idea found it less persuasive than their delusion. This isn't a surprise: the thought of being 'mentally ill' remains so loaded with stigma that most people reject it immediately. So, when it comes to making sense of what is happening to them, individuals often feel stuck between the rock of their delusion and the hard place of mental illness.

But if there's something distinctive about the way people with severe paranoia reason, it's only recently that we've come to understand what's going on. It used to be thought that people with delusions were poorer at logical deduction. For a while it was suggested that delusional thinking stems from difficulty gauging what other people are thinking. In the end, neither of those theories proved persuasive. The evidence was patchy, to say the least. But a big step forward came with the intervention of the clinical psychologist Philippa Garety – who in 1992 became my supervisor at the Institute of Psychiatry. In 1991 Philippa, with her colleagues David Hemsley and Simon Wessely, published a paper that would radically reshape our understanding of the relationship between delusions and reasoning.

Philippa set out to compare the reasoning styles of three different groups: psychiatric patients with delusions; patients with anxiety disorders; and people with no psychiatric disorder. To do that, she asked the participants to take the beads test. It's a simple procedure: all you need is two jars of coloured beads. One jar contains a mix of eighty-five yellow beads and fifteen black beads; the other contains the reverse. The researcher conducting the test chooses a jar and then moves them both out of view. They explain that they are going to take beads, one by one, from a jar and then return them. The participant's task is simply to decide from which of the jars the beads are coming. When they are sure, they tell the researcher. There is no limit on the number of beads they can ask to see before deciding. If they want to inspect all one hundred, so be it.

Philippa discovered that something remarkable happens when people with delusions try the beads task. Remember: there are no prizes for picking a jar quickly. All that matters is that you are certain. Yet 40 per cent of the people with delusions who took part in Philippa's experiment made up their minds after having seen just one bead. Philippa's findings have been replicated repeatedly over the years. As a result, it is now accepted that people with delusions are much more likely to jump to conclusions. They gather much less data before they make their call. It's normally reckoned that a tendency to jump to conclusions

(JTC) is indicated by deciding after having seen no more than two beads. It turns out that around 50 per cent of people with delusions do exactly that. JTC isn't confined to this group, but it is much less common in others. For people without delusions, the figure is around 10 to 20 per cent. JTC has also been found in individuals at high risk of psychosis, and in relatives of people with delusions.

JTC is not confined to people with persistent, long-running delusions. When we compared patients being treated for their very first psychotic episode with a non-clinical population, the patients were twice as likely to jump to conclusions. Again, the more severe the delusion the stronger the tendency to JTC. How those patients fared over the following year also seemed to be influenced by JTC. A year later, those who were still experiencing delusions had all previously scored highly for JTC. In fact, they were twice as likely to have done so as those who had recovered.

How about people with less severely delusional ideas? Are they also more likely to jump to conclusions? It seems so – which fits with the idea that paranoia exists on a spectrum. Some people will be prone to regular, intense and distressing delusions. Others will shrug off the occasional mistrustful feeling. The difference is in the severity and not the essence of the experience. In the first large-scale survey of a non-clinical group, we asked two hundred members of the general public to undertake the beads task. Twenty per cent of the group jumped to a conclusion. And there was something distinctive about that 20 per cent: they were also more likely to believe and be distressed by paranoid thoughts. Interestingly, they weren't more likely to *experience* paranoia. What marked them out was the conviction with which they held these beliefs and, consequently, the impact of those beliefs. (In contrast, when other people experienced paranoid thoughts, they didn't take them seriously. The emotional effect of these thoughts, therefore, was negligible.)

This makes sense: reasoning biases like JTC aren't likely to trigger mistrustful thoughts, but they will determine how we respond to them. We won't, for example, take the time to consider other ways of making sense of our experience. Indeed, in my 2002 survey of one hundred patients with psychosis the two went hand in hand. Given the beads task, the people who jumped to conclusions were also much less likely to suggest an alternative explanation. Those who could offer a range of interpretations asked to see more beads (in other words, gathered more evidence) before forming a view.

Two-four-six

'The human understanding when it has once adopted an opinion . . . draws all things else to support and agree with it. And though there be a greater number and weight of instances to be found on the other side, yet these it either neglects and despises, or else by some distinction sets aside and rejects, in order that by this great and pernicious predetermination the authority of its former conclusions may remain inviolate.'

Francis Bacon, *The New Organon* (1620)

Jumping to conclusions is trivial when the context is a jar of beads. It doesn't matter if your guess is wrong. The stakes in everyday life, on the other hand, can be much higher. This is because JTC results in snap judgements – and snap judgements, being based not on evidence but on our preconceptions, can be misleading. If we're prone to paranoia, those preconceptions can push us into instantly concluding that we are in danger.

Matters are made trickier by the natural human tendency to see what we expect to see. This reflex can be useful – imagine having to weigh up the plausibility of every single proposition. But of course, it can also skew our perception of the world around us. We tend to attach excessive significance to information that appears to confirm our existing beliefs and dismiss data that doesn't. Rather than exploring alternative viewpoints, we prefer to stick with what we know. Psychologists call this the *belief confirmation bias*, and it was neatly demonstrated by the pioneering British cognitive psychologist Peter Wason in 1960. Wason disputed the prevailing view – reaching all the way back to Aristotle – that humans are innately rational beings. His experiments, he argued, 'demonstrate, on a miniature scale, how dogmatic thinking and the refusal to entertain the possibility of alternatives can easily result in error'. In Wason's 2-4-6 task the researcher asks the participant to deduce the rule linking three numbers. The researcher explains that the numbers 2-4-6 conform to the rule. To work it out, the participant can propose other sets of three numbers and the researcher will announce whether they fit the rule.

Now, there's nothing to be gained from going early with a proposed solution. There are no prizes for speed. The objective is accuracy: do whatever it takes to identify the rule. So the participant is encouraged to propose as many sets of numbers as they feel necessary to test their hypotheses. However, most people assume very quickly that the rule is 'numbers increasing by two' and only suggest combinations that do exactly that. They don't try numbers that contradict their hunch. But if human beings were truly natural logicians, this is precisely what they would do. Proving a hypothesis requires more than positive examples. One must try to disprove it (Karl Popper called this the 'falsification principle' and he regarded it as a defining feature of scientific thinking).

As you will have guessed, Wason's rule was not 'numbers increasing by two'. The solution was instead 'any increasing numbers'. People who perform well on the 2-4-6 task generally use three key strategies. First, they tend to suggest sets of numbers that don't fit their hypothesis (they try to 'falsify' their theory). Second, they're open to alternative suggestions. Finally, they don't rush into a declaration, but instead try lots of number sets before coming to a decision. There's a lot of 'cognitive flexibility' here – a readiness to consider alternative interpretations and patiently put them to the test. It's the opposite of what we tend to see in people with paranoid thoughts, or indeed in most individuals.

Slow-Mo

'I don't worry so much, it's my neighbours, they make me stressed and then I'll say "No, I've got to slow down." You have to because if not, if you carry on, you make yourself ill and you'll land up in hospital.'

Neo, the hero of the sci-fi blockbuster *The Matrix*, is equipped with such superhuman reactions that he can evade gunfire, dodging the bullets with ease. To convey Neo's extraordinary powers, the image slows down almost to a stop. (This special effect has become so famous it even has its own name in cinematography: bullet time.) Now, we can track the individual rounds as they glide towards him – and as Neo gracefully swerves to avoid them. The scene seems to me a metaphor for the dizzying flow of thoughts and emotions that life can sometimes entail. And for the desire most of us have sometimes felt to slow down that flow in order to navigate it better.

Arresting the rush of thoughts becomes especially important when it derails us emotionally – when, for example, it makes us feel sad or anxious. This is of course what we're up against with paranoia. And so one of the aims of therapy is to help people manage their thought processes, just as Robert Chapman did so successfully. Rather than hurrying to judgement, we want them to slow down and dodge the bullets of fear and mistrust. We want them to question their paranoid beliefs. We want them to consider alternative explanations for their experience and take the time to weigh up the evidence. We want them, in short, to become more *cognitively flexible*.

This is where the Slow-Mo treatment comes in. Slow-Mo is the product of more than a decade of research. As usual, the treatment we have today is much less the outcome of a single inspirational leap than of numerous painstaking steps. It began as a forty-five-minute PowerPoint session devised in 2010 with Kerry Ross, a doctoral student of Philippa's and mine at the Institute of Psychiatry; was revised and augmented by another of our IoP doctoral students, Helen Waller, a couple of years later; and grew into its current form under the aegis of the talented clinical psychologist Amy Hardy.

> As we navigate our lives, we normally allow ourselves to be guided by impressions and feelings, and the confidence we have in our intuitive beliefs and preferences is usually justified. But not always. We are often confident even when we are wrong, and an objective observer is more likely to detect our errors than we are.

So wrote the celebrated psychologist Daniel Kahneman. What he describes here is *fast thinking*, which is effortless, intuitive and often strongly emotional. It's what we do when we step into the road and suddenly realise that the car we took to be safely in the distance is actually scarily close. It sparks into life when we see the face of a friend. Or when you picked up this book to resume reading. Slow-Mo starts by teaching patients that, although fast thinking is both common and sometimes indispensable – no one should be taking the time to work out whether that car really is likely to hit them – it isn't always helpful. Having learned to spot when they are rushing to judgement unnecessarily, the next step is to *slow down for a moment*. (Sixty per cent of people with severe paranoia find slow, analytic thinking difficult.) Kahneman notes that slow thinking is 'deliberate, effortful, and orderly . . . [and is] often associated with the subjective experience of agency, choice, and concentration'. Once they've hit pause, the person can deploy the techniques they've learned in order to foster that slow thinking: reflecting on their beliefs; brainstorming alternative explanations; weighing up the evidence; and making a choice that allows them to feel and behave more positively.

Slow-Mo is what's known as a 'blended' treatment. It's a mix of in-person sessions with a therapist and computer-based resources: in this case a personalised smartphone app to help patients in between consultations. The app allows patients to record their typical fast thoughts and worries, remind themselves of alternative explanations, and jot down key lessons for the week ahead. Patients told us that they wanted less verbal information and more interactive content. So fast, unhelpful thoughts are depicted as large, grey, rapidly spinning bubbles. The user deals with them by selecting the positive thoughts in slowly rotating coloured bubbles. The fast thoughts shrink as the slow ones grow. These positive thoughts are personalised and always accessible via the app. This makes it much easier for the individual to bring these slower thoughts to mind and, thereby, to feel safer.

With Philippa, Amy, Tom Ward and a large team, we tested Slow-Mo in a randomised controlled trial with 362 patients who had severe paranoia. Slow-Mo helped people reduce their paranoia to a small degree, and it did so by boosting belief flexibility. Just as Robert Chapman discovered, by pushing back on our instinctive reactions to events we gain some distance from our fears. That distance gives us the space in which to think things through. And when that happens, the assumption that other people mean us harm becomes much less plausible:

> I always insisted on going on . . . it might be a split-second decision . . . which is basically fast thinking. I was trained to always look out for the worst-case scenario . . . SlowMo slow thinking wasn't difficult, but it was different . . . I found that using that where I live, all those idiots in the other blocks, if you think through possible other scenarios and then think 'I don't actually know those people and they don't know me, so they can't be talking about me', whereas prior to SlowMo I would think 'Why are they talking about me? What is going on?' and that would stress me out really badly.

Not everyone was comfortable with the technical demands of the phone, but many others found the app invaluable: 'Every day if I go out, I always do what I need to do on it, like take my deep breaths and get me encouraged to go out . . . But that phone is always with me when I'm out.' Some talked about the app as playing the role of a best friend: always there for them, always supportive, always with their welfare at heart. As the weeks went on, though, participants reported not needing to consult the app as often. The therapeutic techniques had become embedded, the lessons learned.

Overall, Slow-Mo's effect on paranoia was modest. But for a few it was dramatic: 'Well the paranoia has dropped quite a bit, yeah. I'm not as extremely paranoid as I used to be.' As their paranoia diminished, patients gradually found themselves able to re-engage with ordinary activities: 'I never used to go out, you see, and I go out on my scooter now with confidence. Before I wouldn't; I always thought people were going to attack me and I don't feel like that now.' It wasn't only paranoia that improved; participants reported positive changes in their all-round mental health. 'It's teaching me to not sort of stress so much. Not, you know, not to get over anxious about stuff'; 'This is the first time in 5 years as I haven't been in hospital with my depression and psychosis. So I think it's really made a difference. Normally I am sort of in hospital three or four months a year.'

Worry

'I'm a worrier but now I'm not a worrier as much as I was . . . it slowed me down quite a lot.'

Slow-Mo trial participant

You can never be quite sure what you're going to find when you trial a treatment. Slow-Mo is all about changing the way people with psychosis reason. But a reviewer of the original grant application suggested we also track its effect on worry (they had seen my earlier worry treatment trial). Rather to our surprise, it turned out to be a canny call. Slow-Mo doesn't only foster cognitive flexibility, it also helps people worry less. And that reduction in worry partly explains the improvements in paranoia.

How do we learn to worry less? Here's (a very abbreviated version of) what I work through with patients – and what I would likely recommend to you too. Worry is all about the worst-case scenario: it's an exceedingly bleak way of looking at the world. But people prone to worry don't tend to see it like this. They may hate the fact that they worry. They may dearly wish they could be free of it. But they also believe that worry helps them. Some people, for example, tell me that worrying allows them to feel that they are in control. Or that it prepares them for problems when they occur. Or that by worrying about something, they can somehow prevent it happening. In fact, worry confers none of these benefits. But the belief produces a vicious cycle. We feel anxious about a situation and respond by worrying about it. But worry redoubles our focus on the worst outcome and thus increases our anxiety. Our worry duly intensifies – and so on. Clearly, we need to break this cycle. For a start, we need to recognise and then evaluate our positive beliefs about worry. What, for instance, are the pros and cons of worry? What would life be like without worry – better or worse? It's useful too to reflect on typical triggers. Are we especially prone to worry at certain times of day, for example, or in specific situations?

Equipped with this insight into how and when worry affects us, we can implement two key techniques to overcome it. The first is to reserve our worrying for a regular daily session – maybe fifteen to thirty minutes. The setting for this 'worry period' should be somewhere private but not comfortable. Sitting on a hard, upright chair at a table is much better than sprawling on the sofa: we don't want worrying to seem relaxing or pleasurable. What if we find ourselves worrying at other times of the day? We stop and save it for later. This is where the second technique comes in. If we know when we're most vulnerable to worry, we can plan activities for those times – activities that are so compelling they leave little mental space for anything else. Exactly what those activities are will vary from person to person. But some have proven especially effective: for example, physical exercise; playing a game or a musical instrument; watching a favourite TV programme or film; speaking to a friend; or practising a mindfulness or relaxation exercise. For all its sophistication, the human mind isn't terribly good at focusing on two things at once. When it comes to reducing worry, this limitation is a boon. All we have to do is discover the activity that can outcompete worry for our attention.

We've known for some years that worry plays an absolutely fundamental role in paranoia – indeed in my view it may well be more influential than reasoning. I saw how worry fuels paranoia for the first time when I met Robert in 1992: the idea that he was in danger nagged away at him night and day. Since then, I've observed it in pretty much every patient I've treated. Four out of five people with persecutory delusions experience the levels of worry seen in patients with generalised anxiety disorder (the mental health condition in which excessive worry is the defining feature). Not only is worry endemic, the more a person worries the more distressing and persistent that paranoia tends to be. It doesn't stop there. As we've come to expect, what is true of people with clinical paranoia also holds for everyday mistrust. If you look for instance at the 2007 Adult Psychiatry Morbidity Survey – which covers a representative sample of over seven thousand adults in England – you'll find that those prone to paranoia are also those who worry most. Remember our virtual London tube train from Chapter 4? Two hundred members of the general population participated in the experiment. None of them had a history of severe mental health problems. Our tube ride prompted paranoia in 40 per cent of the group – and again they were generally also people who worried a lot. These kinds of study don't tell us whether worry causes paranoia. But there are at least a couple of compelling reasons to suggest so.

Consider, for example, the evidence that being a worrier significantly increases the odds that you'll go on to develop paranoia. I analysed data on 2,382 participants in the 2000 British National Psychiatric Morbidity Survey, all of whom had been assessed again eighteen months later. Not only did worriers tend to experience persistent paranoia, reporting it at both the first and follow-up assessments. But people with high levels of worry and no paranoia at the initial interview were much more likely to report it eighteen months later. Then there is the fact that by treating worry we can alleviate paranoia. My 2015 Worry Intervention Trial with 150 patients experiencing persecutory delusions – the first major randomised controlled clinical trial to focus on paranoia and the one that had prompted Slow-Mo's reviewer to suggest we add worry to our battery of assessments – saw a six-week course of worry-focused CBT lead to substantial reductions in the delusions. In fact, fully two-thirds of the decline in paranoia was due to the drop-off in worry.

Why might worry be a contributory cause of paranoia? In this context, worry is an emotional reaction to a paranoid thought. And it's a perfectly understandable one: if I believe like Robert that the government wants me dead, naturally it's going to play on my mind. The problem is that, by repeatedly returning to it, worry keeps that thought alive. Mistrust feeds on the attention it is given. Like some oversized cuckoo in the nest, it crowds out more positive and accurate explanations of what might (or might not) be going on. That only increases the power of paranoid thoughts, making us more fearful, and more worried. So, once again, we have a cycle that needs to be broken. As it happens, Slow-Mo's techniques echo many of those we use when primarily treating worry rather than paranoia. Both teach that, though mistrustful or worried thoughts may seem irresistibly powerful, we can distance ourselves from them. On any given day, we experience many hundreds of thoughts. They're not all accurate. Most are trivial. So, before we let them dictate our feelings and behaviour, it's sensible to test them out. In so doing, as Robert Chapman discovered, we instantly begin to loosen their hold: 'Without doubt, one's delusions are preserved. With doubt, one discovers.'

12.

gameChange

'I was having a lot of problems in terms of confidence around other people. I was very wary about going into certain situations, such as going into crowded places, and that could include cafés, buses, anywhere where there were crowds of people because part of my mental health problems involved being very suspicious about people and what they intended to do. . . . I was always worrying that people were out there to harm me. And for that reason, I shied away from being in social situations as much as I could.'

Tharik, gameChange trial participant

Sometimes things are right in front of you all along. It just takes a while to figure them out. There was so much to learn about paranoia from that first encounter with Robert back in 1992. In some sense, all my work has been about trying to understand what I first observed that rainy autumn day three decades ago. Proust had it right: 'The real voyage of discovery consists not in seeking new landscapes, but in having new eyes.'

One effect of excessive mistrust that I have consistently observed is the distress it causes to those that experience it, and the confusion and worry it brings to those around them. At its extreme, mistrust can bring periods of personal turmoil and

– as we saw in Chapter 6 – damaged relationships. It can play havoc with the fabric of society too, as we will discuss in the next chapter. For Robert, the very first patient I saw, his fear about what others might do to him meant he was rarely able to leave his home. Everyday activities – doing the shopping, using public transport, joining a friend for a coffee – had morphed into superhuman challenges. Hiding away at the back of the house was his defence. I've seen this sort of thing a lot. It's a major reason why, instead of meeting a patient in clinic, home visits are necessary. But only in recent years have I realised that what can seem like an end point – a person ground down by paranoia, too fearful to leave their home alone – must be understood in its own right. It isn't simply the consequence of other difficulties. It is not merely a by-product or a symptom. And it can be directly and successfully treated. I thought I had hit upon a novel and promising way to get that treatment to people. This realisation set in motion a train of consequences.

The usual psychiatric view is that the withdrawal of patients like Robert is a 'negative symptom' of schizophrenia. Consequently, it is bracketed with loss of interest in activities and relationships and difficulty enjoying things, or simply with the marked impairments in functioning that define the presence of a clinical disorder. But it seemed to me that something rather more specific and straightforward might be going on. Robert stayed at home because it felt like the safest place. His paranoia meant he avoided situations in which escape might be difficult. He feared being attacked, but he was also worried that other people would judge him negatively – as shy or awkward or just plain odd. And he was frightened that, if he did venture outside, he wouldn't be able to cope with the intense anxiety he was sure would kick in. In other words, Robert's paranoia, and a whole set of related anxieties, had led to him becoming agoraphobic.

Now agoraphobia – although a distinct disorder with its own

set of clinical criteria – is typically regarded in psychiatry as a kind of secondary manifestation of panic disorder. People avoid going outside because they fear they may experience a panic attack. Agoraphobia and paranoia have therefore inhabited separate theoretical and therapeutic worlds. No one had investigated the links between them. And no one had ever tried to find out how common agoraphobia is in patients like Robert who had been diagnosed with psychosis. So I led the first study, recruiting 1,800 patients attending NHS services. An extraordinary number – two-thirds – showed agoraphobic levels of anxious avoidance. That is, they were so fearful about being out and about that they sought to avoid such situations. But the rate was even higher among the one thousand patients with severe paranoia. Three-quarters of that group experienced clinical levels of agoraphobia.

The great news here is that there is an established remedy for agoraphobic avoidance, though it has never been tested with patients experiencing intense paranoia. (Separate worlds, remember.) It involves the individual working with a therapist to practise going back out into everyday situations. The objective is to discover for themselves that their fears are not an accurate interpretation of what is going on around them. It's a gradual process: step by step, the patient undertakes a series of increasingly challenging activities. This is not something that can be rushed. It takes time for the patient to learn that their fears aren't realistic. Though they may feel anxious, they come to realise that they can handle those feelings. They won't panic, but if they do it doesn't matter. Nothing catastrophic will happen. As you might imagine, patients can find these sessions pretty draining. They are, after all, putting themselves in situations they would normally avoid. Nevertheless, that hard work often brings very substantial rewards. Lives can be transformed.

It is sad then that the number of people with paranoia who

receive this kind of help is tiny, largely because there simply aren't enough clinicians to go around. And it is time-consuming work: rather than a neat one-hour session in the therapist's office, there are trips to the shops, the park, perhaps even a ride on a bus. All in all, mental health services are simply not set up to offer the kind of intervention that could get people who are housebound back into the outside world. Indeed, despite the enthusiasm of patients, carers and NHS England, too few people diagnosed with psychosis receive any significant psychological treatment, whether that's in the consulting room or out of it. So, what to do?

Another day, another grant application

> 'Fiftieth VR Definition: A hint of the experience of life without all the limitations that have always defined personhood.'
>
> Jaron Lanier, *Dawn of the New Everything* (2017)

Like many scientists, I spend more time than I might ideally like putting together funding applications. Detailing what one wants to do and why it is important feels like useful work. But that forms only a small part of most applications, which often run to well over one hundred pages and are largely made up of items such as management and governance plans, itemised budgets, GANTT charts, team CVs, intellectual property strategy . . . Given the research that a successful application makes possible, it would be churlish to complain too much, lovely though it would be to have one's work funded on the strength of a concise email or a strong one-pager. Nevertheless, assembling a major grant application takes many months of collaborative effort. And when you've finally submitted one, the prospect of immediately beginning work on another is distinctly unappealing – especially if you're feeling confident about your chances with the first. So when in 2017, less than twenty-four hours after pressing the submit button, I was told about a new award sponsored by the UK National Institute for Health and Care Research, I decided to let it pass. That I changed my mind was largely due to the persuasion of John Geddes, my head of department, who seemed to think the NIHR's new funding competition – the Invention for Innovation (i4i) Mental Health Challenge Award – was right up my street. As it turned out, he had a point. (And I was wrong to be confident about the other application, much to my continued irritation.)

The i4i award supports the development of medical technologies – and not just their development but, assuming all goes to plan and the product is both clinically beneficial and cost-effective, preparation for rollout in the NHS. What, you may be wondering, does a clinical psychologist know about medical technology? Isn't mental health care an inherently analogue affair: two people face to face discussing thoughts, feelings and behaviours? In fact, the i4i competition reflects a growing awareness that digital products have an important role to play in treating psychological problems. An in-person meeting with a therapist can be hugely beneficial, of course. But that doesn't mean other strategies can't also work. Mental health care isn't a zero-sum game. It's implausible to think that seeing a therapist is the only way to tackle the psychological factors that cause difficulties. It also doesn't get us very far in practical terms: as we've noted, there is a shortage of therapists. Besides, not everyone feels comfortable with the in-person approach.

Over the past twenty years I've explored the contribution that digital technology, and in particular virtual reality (VR), can make both to understanding why psychological problems occur and to treating them. (We've explored some of this work in earlier chapters.) In that time, I've become increasingly convinced that VR interventions need not be an inferior substitute for the 'real thing' of face-to-face therapy. Rather, they can be highly effective treatments in their own right. Indeed, it seems to me that VR is an inherently therapeutic medium: safe, compelling, and perfectly suited to experiential learning. What is more, VR can help us jump the hurdle of the shortage of therapists. There is an awful lot at stake here. If we can automate the treatment – in other words, embed the therapy in the VR – we can begin to envisage a world in which everyone with access to, say, the internet (and of course there is a long way to go before even that objective is attained) can get the mental health care they need. Maybe, I reflected, the i4i scheme offered an opportunity to try to begin building that future for people with severe paranoia.

The idea was a simple one: give NHS patients with psychosis who have agoraphobic symptoms the chance to explore immersive replicas of everyday situations. Guided by a virtual therapist, they could practise new and more productive ways of thinking, feeling and behaving in those situations. Gradually, and encouraged by the virtual therapist, out would go the defensive strategies: no avoiding the situation, no reticence about eye contact, no reliance on someone else always being there as protection. Grade the situations by difficulty so that users can become comfortable in increasingly challenging scenarios. And do whatever we could to make the program easy to use, engaging, and even entertaining too.

As is the way of these things, the application was drafted, redrafted and drafted again. Having made it through the first round of the competition, yet more drafting was required. That second application took us on to the shortlist and an interview and presentation. Finally, in February 2018, we learned that we had won the inaugural i4i Mental Health Challenge Award. We celebrated, naturally. For one evening. And then the next day we got to work. There was no time to lose. We had said we could design a new treatment, program it in virtual reality, prepare services to use the treatment, test it, do the health economics and plan a rollout – all in three years. It was ambitious, for sure. But mental health care deserves ambition.

Designing gameChange

'. . . to play implies a reduction in the seriousness of the consequences of errors and of setbacks. . . . It is, in a word, an activity that is for itself and not for others. It is, in consequence, a superb medium for exploration. Play provides a courage all its own.'

Jerome Bruner, psychologist

Every project, unfortunately, needs a name. I say unfortunately because in my experience at least, choosing that name can be a peculiarly arduous task – one not made any easier when you consider that you're going to have to live with the outcome for, in some cases, several years. Ideas are painfully extracted from collaborators and consultants; suggestions are kicked around; contradictory preferences are expressed; a decision, at last, is arrived at. But this time around I was sure we'd got it right, and quickly too. 'gameChange' encapsulated the transformative ambition of what we aimed to produce, its incarnation as a computer program, and the playfulness we wanted to build into the experience.

The name was also popular with our patient panel. We wouldn't have chosen it if they'd felt differently. Today it is increasingly recognised that mental health research ought not to be something 'done to' patients. Instead, people with lived experience are essential collaborators and colleagues. For several

years now I have had the pleasure of working with Dr Thomas
Kabir at the McPin Foundation, a charity which believes that
effective mental health care requires the expertise of people
affected by mental health problems. McPin convened a
gameChange Lived Experience Advisory Panel (LEAP)
comprising ten people with lived experience of psychosis. The
LEAP was to prove critical in the design of the treatment. They
helped define the VR scenarios; they fed into the design of
characters; advised on what the virtual coach should say; tested
the evolving VR prototypes; and helped craft a questionnaire
to assess how easy and engaging the program was for patients
to use. And of course they played a key part in naming the
project. In addition to the LEAP's myriad contributions, we
held a dozen design workshops involving people with lived
experience. All in all, fifty-three people with lived experience
contributed to the design of gameChange, with over 500 hours
of input.

The outcome of this process, which also included several
workshops with NHS staff, was a plan for a VR experience that
would take patients into six everyday situations: stepping out
of a front door onto a busy street; getting on to a bus; and
visiting a GP surgery, a convenience store, a coffee shop and a
pub. In each of those situations, users were invited to progress
through five levels, each a little more challenging than the last.
So, for example, the first level of each situation would be relatively quiet, with few people around. As the patient became
more confident, the scenes would grow steadily busier. We'd
ratchet up the anxiety in other ways too, adding CCTV cameras,
hooded teenagers and police officers, and positioning characters
closer to the patient or blocking the exit. Always the aim was
for users to learn that, even in situations that seemed really
frightening, they were in fact safe. And to use those new memories of safety to counteract ingrained thoughts of danger.

But the patient wasn't to be merely a bystander in these situations. At every level they would be asked to perform a task. Because of course we don't glide through the world as invisible observers: we act in that world. There are journeys we must make, chores to accomplish, people with whom we wish to communicate. And so, among many other activities, our patients would order a coffee in a café, give their name to a GP receptionist, meet a friend in a pub full of football fans, wait on the street for a taxi, and buy provisions in a convenience store. These activities weren't chosen at random. They reflected the kind of situations and interactions that so many people with psychosis find difficult. To spice it up – to add elements of the unexpected and even the ridiculous – we included playful activities such as bursting the bubbles blown by a toddler in a buggy or catching leaflets jumbled into the air by a fan. Partly the point was to increase the fun quotient. But there was also a therapeutic angle:

> [There are] little games inside of it, like in the GP reception office a fan gets switched on and you have to grab papers. There's a little child in a buggy and one of them blowing bubbles and you have to pop them. Which is just silly fun but it's also that totally unexpected, totally out of the blue, and yet you cope with it. So it's helping you prepare for life, the unexpected. (Danny)

When a patient stretches to burst a bubble they make themselves the centre of attention. Moreover, their movement takes them closer to the other characters. In doing so, they abandon the defensive behaviour that so often keeps patients, when they do enter public spaces, on the margins. Instead, and sometimes before they realise it, they are drawn into the fray. They participate; they join in; they get things done.

'Hi – I'm Nic'

What would your ideal therapist look like? Players of computer games are used to defining the gender, ethnicity, age, physical appearance and personality of the avatars that accompany them through their adventures. We would have loved to do the same in gameChange. One day I hope we shall. But the programming demands, and therefore the cost, of doing this in VR at the time meant that we had to settle on one character. That character is Nic (short for Now I Can, a previous result of a long branding process . . .).

Getting Nic right was a big deal. After all, she was going to guide our users through the program as a more or less constant companion and source of advice, encouragement and support. A member of the LEAP put it this way:

> [Nic is] not just the person who is providing instructions, it is the person who is there to reassure, not about the facts she is saying, but the trust part. Yes, it's about having someone who is there for you in any situation, not someone who spouts facts at you. It's about not being alone, a sense of bond, understanding and care.

The Nic patients meet in gameChange is a white woman in her thirties with short auburn hair. She is fairly slim, of average height, and soberly dressed in olive green trousers and brown jacket. But she didn't always look like this. Sketches produced by character artists were mulled over at design meetings. Successive revisions edged us ever closer to the finished article. Nic gradually took shape in our 3D realm.

Yet Nic isn't simply a visual presence in gameChange. She is also the voice of the experience. In many ways, that voice is more important than her appearance. This is because immersive VR is not solely a visual medium. Users are much more than passive spectators. We don't watch a VR scenario as we might watch a movie; we inhabit it. gameChange's users were likely to focus far more on the scene around them, and their tasks within it, than on Nic. But though they might only look at her sporadically, they were much more likely to listen to her, to be guided, encouraged and advised by her. With this in mind, we wanted Nic's voice to be friendly but also calm and authoritative. So it was time for another selection process, and this time not from sketches of fictional characters but from voice actor audition reels. Our choice was Helen Jessica Liggat, whose gentle Edinburgh accent we hoped would have the added advantage – at least for the patients in our English project sites – of being relatively unburdened by preconceptions and prior associations.

Early in 2019 Helen came to our VR lab in Oxford to record the script, which by now ran to more than a hundred pages and had been repeatedly role-played and reviewed over the previous weeks. The recording process was a little different to Helen's previous assignments. We weren't simply taping her voice. We were also filming her movements in order to animate Nic in a realistic fashion. Poor Helen gamely spent three long, coffee-fuelled days encased in a motion capture suit – an outfit that resembles a wetsuit, with matching hat, gloves and shoes, all studded with sensors beaming back data to the studio's infrared cameras. She was joined in her ordeal by two other professional actors, who between them voiced the numerous minor characters in the scenarios. (As they say in radio drama credits: other parts were played by members of the cast . . .)

When at last the sessions were over, the mocap suits back on the clothes rail, and the actors on the train home, the programming team began the laborious task of processing hundreds of audio and visual files, selecting the most successful takes, cleaning up the sound (who knew there were so many planes, helicopters and emergency vehicles?), and mapping Helen's speech and movements on to the face and body of Nic. It was the last piece in the VR puzzle – taking its place among the carefully crafted environments and minutely choreographed sequence of user activities. After a few weeks of in-house testing, we were ready to see whether gameChange could really make a difference to people with severe paranoia.

The trial

'From this evening I must give the British people a very simple instruction – you must stay at home.'
                              Boris Johnson, 23 March 2020

A clinical trial of gameChange's size, duration and technological complexity is a mammoth undertaking. Nine NHS trusts. Hundreds of patients. Eighteen months from first patient recruitment to final follow-up. Indeed, we were embarking on the largest ever trial of a virtual reality treatment for mental health problems. Across our five sites – in Newcastle, Manchester, Nottingham, Bristol and Oxfordshire – we aimed to recruit 432 participants. From a standing start in July 2019 things were moving along pretty well. And then Covid-19 hit. As UK readers will remember vividly, on 23 March 2020 the prime minister announced that the country was entering lockdown. The trial came to an abrupt halt. And we had no idea when it might be able to restart.

The weeks ticked by. I remained at home, trying to manage via Zoom a project that had been turned upside down. At long last, after six months of near stasis, in September 2020 we began treating patients again. Even once we got going, however, complications abounded. For one thing, we had to change the way we measured patient progress given that face-to-face assessments were now prohibited by the NHS trusts. For another, routine cleanliness was no longer sufficient; now the VR equipment had to be painstakingly decontaminated after each session. (I won't go into the details here, but the process involved eight steps and industrial quantities of detergent wipes.) Then there was the fact that we were encouraging patients to engage with everyday activities at precisely the time when the authorities were advising the public to avoid being around other people. Could a treatment for agoraphobia possibly gain any sort of therapeutic traction in the face of constant warnings about the dangers of going outside? And how could patients take what they'd learned in VR into real-life situations, given that so many of those situations were now off limits?

We persevered. Half our patients were randomly allocated to receive the VR therapy, plus their existing treatment – which generally meant antipsychotic medication, regular visits from a community mental health worker, and occasional outpatient appointments with a psychiatrist. The other 50 per cent of the group simply carried on with their existing treatment. We assessed our participants before they began the trial, immediately after they had completed the six-week VR therapy, and then again six months later. What we were mainly interested in was the degree to which they avoided everyday social situations and the amount of distress they felt in those situations. To help us understand this, Sinéad Lambe, myself and team developed the Oxford Agoraphobic Avoidance Scale (see Table 5):

Table 5

Do you feel you could do this right now?	Yes, I could do this now	No, I'd get too anxious	How anxious would you feel doing this?
			No distress (0) 1 2 3 4 Moderate distress (5) 6 7 8 9 Extreme distress (10)
1. Stand outside your home on your own for 5 minutes.			0 1 2 3 4 5 6 7 8 9 10
2. Walk down a quiet street on your own.			0 1 2 3 4 5 6 7 8 9 10
3. Walk down a busy street with someone you know.			0 1 2 3 4 5 6 7 8 9 10
4. Travel on your own on the bus for several stops.			0 1 2 3 4 5 6 7 8 9 10
5. Sit in the waiting room of your GP/ health centre on your own for 5 minutes.			0 1 2 3 4 5 6 7 8 9 10
6. Purchase an item in a local shop from a shop assistant.			0 1 2 3 4 5 6 7 8 9 10
7. Go to a shopping centre on your own for 15 minutes.			0 1 2 3 4 5 6 7 8 9 10
8. Sit in a café on your own for 10 minutes.			0 1 2 3 4 5 6 7 8 9 10

As you can see, the scale measures both avoidance and distress. For the former, scores can range from 0 to 8, with 3–5 being high and 6–8 severe. Distress scores can be anything from 0 to 80. We categorise a score of 46–65 as indicating high distress and anything above that as severe distress.

We also tracked whether the patients fared differently depending on whether they had been supported in the VR therapy by an assistant psychologist, CBT therapist, or peer support worker (that is, someone with their own lived experience of mental health problems). These staff members are there to assist in setting up the hardware, explain what is going to happen, and help organise homework to consolidate the learning from VR. Essentially, it's about ensuring the patient takes the very most they can from the treatment. A crucial role then, but not one that need be performed by a clinical psychologist or psychiatrist. Or at least, that was my hypothesis.

'Another world': The patient experience

When done properly, virtual reality is a curiously paradoxical experience. At one level, you know very well that what you see and hear is an illusion. And at another, it feels entirely real: 'Going into VR was like going into another world, kind of thing. It was really like everything was not realistic, you could tell it was all fake, but at the same time you felt like you were actually in there.'

That double take is therapeutically critical. First because it means that people will attempt things in VR that they would avoid in real life: 'Because it was VR, it was always in the back of your mind, "I'm safe, I can take this off at any time." But it was so immersive it felt real. So it was that perfect middle ground of doing these things while not being thrown into it and thinking "Oh my god, I've got to run, people are going to judge us." If you do panic, you can just take the headset off.' And second because it allows the lessons learned in the virtual world to be useful in the real world.

One of the great merits of VR is the opportunity it provides for patients to be appropriately challenged. I want patients to leave their comfort zone. I want them to test themselves. But not beyond what they can handle. As one participant put it: 'It's a fine line: you want it to be realistic enough, so it's a good practice, but it's also quite helpful if it's not totally realistic because then you get that security of knowing that it's not real.' It's not always a comfortable experience: 'I really enjoyed it. Well, I say enjoyed it, it was actually quite hard work. I found it very realistic when I went in, more than I expected, I think. And it was a lot harder than I thought it was going to be.'

As we had hoped, gameChange provided participants with a safe place to practise new ways of behaving in everyday situations – and to take those innovations into the real world:

> The everyday situations that I found difficult, the more I practised them in the VR, the more I could get confident and be more confident in day-to-day life. I think because I was learning about it in the VR and practising and practising and practising, I could then take that and build up more confidence and do it in the everyday real world. (Joy)

> What I tried to do is, when I'd had the VR sessions, I tried to use the sort of techniques that I'd learned and the lessons, if you like, that I'd learned during those particular sessions in the real world as a practice. So on one occasion I got onto a bus, sat down, and I ended up chatting to a lady on the bus and we were chatting so much that I forgot to get off! I felt so confident on that bus. (Tharik)

These patients were dropping their defences. They weren't avoiding the situations that triggered their paranoid and anxious thoughts. They weren't trying simply to get through the experience as quickly and unobtrusively as possible. They were immersing themselves in this strange new reality and discovering the disjunction between what they expected and what in fact transpired: 'It's kind of like relearning confidence . . . and putting memories of situations that are good and okay and just normal into my, you know, memory bank rather than the awful things that I was imagining were going to happen.'

The trial results

As it happens, more than half a century ago one of the very first randomised controlled trials of psychological therapy was that of a treatment for severe agoraphobia. In 1966, Michael Gelder (who in 1969 became Oxford's first Professor of Psychiatry and set up the department where I worked until 2023) and Isaac Marks carried out a small trial with twenty patients, three-quarters of whom had been unable to leave their home unaccompanied. The results proved disappointing to Gelder and Isaacs. Only four out of ten patients showed good improvements. Moreover, the demands on patients and therapists alike were immense: sixty sessions of face-to-face behaviour therapy provided over six months.

Most gameChange patients, by contrast, completed the treatment in just six sessions, with around three hours spent in VR. That was enough to see significant improvement. Agoraphobic avoidance decreased. So did distress. Not everyone made gains. For patients with lower levels of anxiety, who were able to go out locally, and perhaps struggled with complex social interactions, there was less evidence for treatment benefit. But the patients that made the most progress were generally those in the most acute need: the people who found it hardest to leave home, the people with the highest levels of mental health symptoms. And for these patients gameChange also delivered a reduction in paranoia. Of course, I want everyone to benefit from gameChange. That said, if I had to choose a group of patients for whom the treatment would be life-changing, it would be those with the severest mental health problems.

The trial results showed that gameChange can be delivered by a range of mental health workers. It certainly doesn't require, say, a clinical psychologist. This was a big win. Because it suggests that, suitably trained, a very wide range of staff can help deliver gameChange: assistant psychologists, CBT therapists, peer support workers, and in the future other mental health professionals such as occupational therapists and support workers. At a stroke, the number of staff members available to provide psychological therapy is thus dramatically increased. And because headsets are rapidly becoming both cheaper and easier to use, we can begin to envisage patients taking the kit home with them and practising whenever they like. Of course, it doesn't much matter how effective a treatment is, nor how easy it is to deploy, if patients don't like it. But all the evidence suggests that gameChange was a positive experience for the trial participants. Uptake was high and feedback consistently enthusiastic. We've seen a similar response with our other VR therapies: tech really does seem to entice people into treatment and keep them coming back for more.

What next?

Many research projects in mental health show promise. Indeed, they sometimes produce amazing results for the relatively small groups of people who experience them in clinical trials. Yet all too frequently the story ends there. Delivering a new treatment, however effective, to patients at scale remains an exceptional event. And so I am taking nothing for granted with gameChange. Nevertheless, as I write this there are good reasons to be optimistic. We have a treatment that will bring real benefits to patients with some of the most challenging mental health difficulties. And it will do so without costing services a fortune. Several NHS trusts have committed to using the program. Others are close. Meanwhile, gameChange is taking its first small steps in the US and other countries.

gameChange can be delivered in patients' homes and in community mental health clinics. But it might also make a huge difference on in-patient psychiatric wards. These are facilities where psychological therapy is rare and boredom high: 'All you did was just sitting around, and there was nothing for you to do . . . no program to keep you busy . . . it's not good . . . I stagnate.' gameChange could be especially helpful in preparing patients to return to the outside world. Patients tend to be very vulnerable after discharge, resulting in high rates of relapse and readmission. And if VR headsets were accessible on wards, additional, freely available VR programs such as physical activity games, relaxation and meditation exercises could also be used by patients as therapeutic activities that reduce boredom and enhance recovery.

While writing this book, I have often thought of Robert and wondered how he is faring now. I hope that he has managed to recover from his paranoia and other problems, that he has been able to get his life back on track. But I know it is possible that he is still hiding away at home, a prisoner of his fears. I wonder what he would make of gameChange. Would he find it helpful? Could it have changed things around for him as dramatically as it has done for many people in our trial? And are we finally reaching a point when everyone with the kind of problems experienced by Robert can access treatments like gameChange?

Literally, it has changed my life, it has turned us around. I'm literally going out, enjoying myself on the beach and stuff, having a day out in nice sunny weather. These are things I couldn't face before gameChange. So, if someone's where I was, I just hope they can get what I got out of it. (Tharik)

13.

Oceans of mistrust

*'Covid-19 is the greatest test that we have faced together
since the formation of the United Nations.'*
António Guterres, UN Secretary General

*'In my understanding, the destructive power of this virus
is overestimated. Maybe it's even being promoted for
economic reasons.'*
Jair Bolsonaro, former president of Brazil 2019–22

Lockdown, as we saw in the previous chapter, brought the
gameChange trial to an abrupt halt. The enforced hiatus
prompted a return to a topic that had been on my mind periodically for over a decade. (Looking back, I think it helped me
cope with the oddness of the times, and the challenges of trying
to keep existing research projects moving forwards during the
chaos of a pandemic.) Because Covid-19 infections weren't the
only thing proliferating in early 2020. So too were conspiracy
theories about the virus. Some were propagated by highly influential sources; some emerged from obscure pockets of the
internet. They included the ideas that the pandemic was a hoax;
that the virus had been deliberately created by the Chinese
government, the Russian government, the US government,
'Zionists', the Gates Foundation or the Canadian National

Microbiology lab (from where it had been stolen by Chinese researchers); that it was linked to the rollout of 5G wireless technology; and that a vaccine was unnecessary given that infection could be prevented or cured by the consumption of oregano oil, vitamin C, bananas, garlic, salt water, alcohol, hot drinks, bleach, cocaine or camel urine. I could go on. These ideas mushroomed so rapidly that as early as February 2020 the World Health Organization was already warning of an 'infodemic' in which 'an over-abundance of information . . . makes it hard for people to find trustworthy sources and reliable guidance when they need it'. This was, of course, precisely the moment when many of us – until then blithely ignorant about the virus – were starting to seek out that guidance. The stakes, according to WHO Director General Tedros Adhanom Ghebreyesus, could hardly have been higher: 'People must have access to accurate information to protect themselves and others. At the World Health Organization we're not just battling the virus, we're also battling the trolls and conspiracy theories that undermine our response. Misinformation on the coronavirus might be the most contagious thing about it.'

Conspiracy beliefs had long intrigued me – which, I guess, as a paranoia researcher is hardly a surprise. Like paranoia, what we're seeing with conspiracy thinking is a form of excessive mistrust. Like paranoia, conspiracy theories are an attempt to make sense of puzzling, unsettling or threatening events. It's worth noting too that 'conspiracy theory' – again like 'paranoia' – can be a somewhat fuzzy term: one we all use but not necessarily to mean the same thing. For clarity, then, I define a conspiracy theory as a belief that the world, or an event, is not as it seems to be. It is suspected that the truth has been covered up by those in positions of authority. Finally, for all the conviction with which it may be held, a conspiracy theory will fail a proof test: it isn't backed up by evidence. Of course, almost by definition it can be difficult to know whether there is a conspiracy afoot. Things are made tougher by the fact that, as we all know, those with power do sometimes seek to mislead. So, although I take the view that true conspiracy theories are unhelpful, neither do I advocate a Pollyannaish acceptance of whatever we are told. We should be vigilant, we should question, and above all we should be guided by the evidence. (Of course, as we'll see below, gauging the reliability of the evidence has become arguably more difficult than ever.)

In 2020 little research had been done on the psychology of conspiracy theories. I suspect the neglect stemmed from an assumption that conspiracy theories were confined to a handful of credulous eccentrics and, as such, unworthy of scientific attention. Indeed, soon after arriving in Oxford in 2011 I assembled a great multidisciplinary team spanning several universities in order to study the biological, cognitive and social causes of conspiracy beliefs. The funding bodies, however, weren't interested. One interview took place on my birthday, but no gifts were forthcoming. Instead, what I left with was the impression that the topic had been deemed too 'niche'. But I'd been down that road with paranoia and knew that such assumptions could be spectacularly wrong. So, with the clinical psychologist Richard Bentall, in 2016 I analysed responses to a nationally representative survey of US adults carried out a few years earlier. (The survey had focused on the prevalence of mental health problems; among the dozens of questions, I'd spotted an interesting one that had never been analysed.) Though the survey predated the ubiquity of social media and the 'post-truth' culture fomented by, for instance, the Trump presidency, more than a quarter (26.7 per cent) of the 5,645 participants had endorsed the statement: 'I am convinced there is a conspiracy behind many things in the world.' These people were more likely to be male, unmarried and poor. They also tended to be less educated, from an ethnic minority group, and to regard themselves as of lower social standing than others. Often, they weren't in great physical or psychological shape. They were more likely to think about suicide, felt less secure in their relationships, and lacked robust social networks. Unsurprisingly, then, they were more likely to meet the criteria for a psychiatric condition. All in all, what we found supported what other researchers had previously discovered: conspiracy beliefs flourish particularly among people who, in diverse ways, exist on the margins of society. But there was more. Those who were receptive to the conspiracy belief also generally answered yes to the question: 'Did you ever believe that there was an unjust plot going on to harm you or to have people follow you that your family and friends did not believe was true?' In other words, these people were not just susceptible to conspiracy beliefs. They were also given to paranoia. Though the two are definitely distinct phenomena, paranoia and conspiracy theories have much in common too. They are links in a chain of suspicion, manifestations of an ingrained mistrust. And, judging by the US data at least, there was a great deal of that mistrust around.

How prevalent, I wondered in March 2020 as the world ground to a standstill, were Covid-19 conspiracy theories? They drew a lot of media coverage, for sure, but were they actually believed by significant numbers of people? (I doubted it but at that point who knew?) And what could we learn about the people who espoused these ideas? Would their demographic and psychological profile match what we'd observed in the US group? These were not merely academic questions. On the contrary, a very great deal hung on the outcome. Because if there had been a time when conspiracy theorists could be discounted as mere cranks (and I doubt it was ever really sensible), that time was long behind us. One has only to think back to the publication in 1998 of Andrew Wakefield's notorious paper on the measles, mumps and rubella (MMR) vaccine. In the UK, the vaccine is typically made available to children in two doses, one at twelve months and the second at around forty months; although soon refuted, Wakefield's suggestion that it could cause autism and colitis led to a dramatic fall in the number of children vaccinated. Uptake of the initial dose in the UK plummeted from 95 per cent (the target set by the World Health Organization to maintain herd immunity) in 1995 to around 80 per cent in 2003, leading to a sharp rise in cases of measles. In July 2023 the UK Health Security Agency warned that London was at risk of a major measles outbreak, with MMR first-dose vaccination rates down to 69.5 per cent in some parts of the city. (It's worth remembering how serious these illnesses can be. In 2017 110,000 people died from measles globally. In 1990, prior to extensive vaccination campaigns, the figure was 872,000.) Even more damagingly, doubts about the MMR vaccine have fed a suspicion that *all* vaccines may be dangerous, and that the governments and scientists who promote their use cannot be trusted.

And yet of course vaccination programmes depend on uptake. Our choice is personal; the implications of our decision are far broader. If we can treat enough people, formerly lethal diseases can be all but eradicated. Fall short, on the other hand, and a virus or other pathogen will continue to circulate. By March 2020 it was clear that a comprehensive vaccination programme would necessarily form a key part of the response to the pandemic. But it was also obvious that a vaccine was, at best, many months away. In the meantime, we would have to rely on lockdown precautions. Like a vaccination programme, the success of those lockdown measures was dependent on trust. High-profile interventions by the police made the headlines, but we were all reliant on the people around us to keep contact to a minimum, isolate when ill with the virus, and in due course to come forward for vaccination. And in order for all that to happen, the public needed to trust the advice of ministers and the scientific consensus on which it was based.

So, I wondered, how robust was that trust in 2020? Crucially, could it affect how likely people were to follow the lockdown guidance? To find out, in May our team swiftly put together the Oxford Coronavirus Explanations, Attitudes and Narratives Survey – OCEANS – quizzing 2,500 adults in England, selected to be representative of the country as a whole on a number of factors such as age, gender, ethnicity, income and region. Members of my research team trawled the internet, bravely descending into many murky rabbit holes, to assemble a long list of Covid-19 conspiracy beliefs. A survey firm collected the data, which arrived on the evening of 11 May. By the following day I had written up the results and submitted the paper for publication. The results were so unsettling that getting the word out seemed like it ought not to wait. I had predicted that perhaps one in twenty (5 per cent) of the participants would express support for the extreme Covid-19 conspiracy beliefs listed in our questionnaire. I was mistaken – very mistaken. One in five people, for example, considered it possible that the virus had been created by Jews in order to destroy the global economy. A quarter were receptive to the idea that Covid-19 had been manufactured by the United Nations and World Health Organization in order to take control. Twenty per cent thought that Bill Gates could be behind it all and a similar percentage suspected the virus was a hoax. Asked whether the pandemic was a deliberate attempt to reduce the global population, around 40 per cent were at least partially in agreement. Was lockdown a ruse to impose mass surveillance? Forty per cent believed it might be. Almost half of our participants endorsed to some degree the idea that 'Coronavirus is a bioweapon developed by China to destroy the West'. A similar proportion thought the mainstream media could be deliberately feeding the public misinformation about the virus and lockdown. All in all, just 50 per cent of those we surveyed unequivocally rejected every one of the conspiracy beliefs we put to them. A quarter showed a consistent pattern of conspiracy thinking.

People in OCEANS tended not to endorse just one conspiracy belief. This was not single-issue scepticism: it was generalised suspicion of those in authority. This sometimes had the curious effect of leading individuals to endorse contradictory ideas. So, for example, those who saw lockdown as a plot by environmental activists also felt that 'globalists' seeking to destroy religion might be behind it. (Other research has found similar patterns, for example that people are able to believe both that Princess Diana faked her own death *and* that she was murdered, and that Osama bin Laden is still alive *and* that he was already dead when US special forces entered his compound in May 2011.) Our Covid-19 doubters were dubious about human-induced climate change. And they were unconvinced by the idea of vaccination in general. Around 16 per cent of people in our survey believed, at least to some extent, that vaccination safety data are often fabricated; that the authorities are covering up the harm that immunisation can cause children; and that the government is hiding a link between vaccination and autism. Another 20–25 per cent of respondents were neutral in their opinion – they were, in other words, sitting on the fence. This means that only around two-thirds of people rejected these conspiracy beliefs. Thirty per cent thought that the search for a coronavirus vaccine was probably unnecessary because a remedy already existed. That remedy, they believed, was being withheld by the World Health Organization.

Our findings were published on 19 May 2020. They were not to everyone's taste. Perhaps because the data were so unpalatable, we were accused of exaggerating the prevalence of conspiracy thinking. But OCEANS demonstrated that mistrust was not an abstraction. Nor was it marginal. On the contrary, this degree of suspicion risked derailing the effort to combat coronavirus. Today, the memory of the first few weeks and months of the pandemic – the fear, uncertainty, and bewildering sense of dislocation so many of us felt – may have dimmed. So it's worth recalling that, by the beginning of May 2020, almost thirty thousand people in the UK had died from the virus. (This was just nine weeks after the country's first reported death. Ten days later the figure had risen to forty thousand.) Every day around a thousand people were being admitted to hospital with Covid-19. Schools, and many businesses, closed indefinitely. Most of the UK population was required to spend virtually every hour at home, avoiding social contact and only venturing out for essential supplies and one exercise session. Yet those in our survey who endorsed conspiracy thinking tended to be dismissive of public health guidance on Covid-19. They were less likely, for example, to stay at home. They frequently rejected the idea that they should stay two metres apart from other people, wash their hands or wear a face mask. They wouldn't use a contact tracing app, nor take a Covid test. And when a vaccine was eventually rolled out, they said they'd be reluctant to accept it. They were also much more likely to report paranoia – in other words, these were often people given to mistrust in general. They were frequently, though not inevitably, hypervigilant both to societal threats *and* danger to themselves personally.

Why was such a large proportion of the public so suspicious of the scientific consensus on Covid-19? Well, the pandemic seems to me to have arrived at a time when trust was already under growing pressure. In part this reflects a lack of social cohesion. Research suggests that conspiracy beliefs are more common in – though certainly not confined to – people who are socially disadvantaged. That the number of the 'left behind' has increased in the UK over recent decades is indicated by rising rates of inequality. (The same is true of the US.) If you believe that those in positions of authority are careless about your welfare you might well treat their pronouncements on Covid-19 (and pretty much everything else) with scepticism. Mistrust, as we have seen throughout this book, builds on feelings of vulnerability. It is rooted in anxiety about what the future may hold. Those who are marginalised are almost by definition vulnerable. They are more likely to face adversity – for example, poverty, ill health (physical and mental) and discrimination – and less well-placed to cope with it.

Indeed, some groups are acutely aware of having been the victims of actual conspiracies involving the medical profession. Although black Americans have been twice as likely to die from Covid-19 as non-Hispanic white Americans, they have been less willing to come forward for vaccination. Part of the explanation is what happened at Tuskegee. In 1932, researchers in Alabama began to study the effects of untreated syphilis on black sharecroppers, most of them illiterate and all of them poor. The sharecroppers were not informed about the true nature of the study, nor that they had syphilis. Instead, they were told that they were suffering the effects of 'bad blood'. When penicillin became available in the 1940s, syphilis became suddenly treatable. But not in Tuskegee, where those in the study were both denied treatment and prevented from seeking it elsewhere. As Talha Burki has written: 'The researchers simply watched them die, and then examined their bodies.' The study was closed down in 1972 after an investigation by the Associated Press. By then, many of the unwitting participants had died from syphilis.

Tuskegee was not an isolated incident – the forced sterilisation of black women in the US in the twentieth century is just one further example of egregious medical discrimination – but it has become emblematic. Reed Tucker, a community leader with the Black Coalition Against Covid-19, noted:

> The number one rate-limiting step for me, in terms of engaging with the Black community in the fight against AIDS, was Tuskegee . . . All these decades later, and Tuskegee has still been a huge obstacle when it comes to engaging the Black community in the fight against Covid-19. Tuskegee is an institutionalised memory. It exists in our minds and culture as a proxy for a much larger set of feelings and emotions, things to do with the racist way Black communities have been treated by the institutions of this country.

But Covid-19 scepticism isn't simply part of the long tail of decades of inequality and discrimination. Into the mix too must go the recent aggressive challenge to conventional notions of truth and those who have traditionally communicated it. It's the wave Michael Gove was riding back in 2016 when he declared during the Brexit campaign that 'people in this country have had enough of experts'. It's what Donald Trump is still stoking when he insists, for instance, that Joe Biden fraudulently won the 2020 US presidential election. It is a world of 'alternative facts' in which we are encouraged to select the reality that most closely conforms to our feelings about how the world should be. Facilitating this wild ride of relativism is of course the advent of the internet and the ubiquity of social media. Estimates suggest that the average adult in the UK now spends around an hour and fifty minutes on social media each day. In the US, surveys put the figure at around two hours ten minutes. Among younger people, that figure is likely to be very much higher. Moreover, we're not merely sharing holiday photos or finalising arrangements for Friday night. Oxford's Reuters Institute for the Study of Journalism noted in June 2022 that data from forty-six countries across six continents showed social media becoming increasingly important as a source of news. That is especially so for the 18–24 age group who aren't simply more likely to go online for news: 'they are much less likely to visit a traditional news website or to pay for online news – and they are often wary of giving up their data. Deeply networked, they are increasingly accessing news in video or audio on networks like Instagram, TikTok, YouTube, or Spotify.' The Reuters Institute also found a good deal of scepticism about the reliability of news providers. In the UK only 34 per cent thought they could trust the news most of the time. In the US, the figure was just 26 per cent (the lowest of the countries surveyed and on a par with Taiwan and Slovakia). Increased diversity in the voices we can hear is clearly a good thing, but who guarantees the credibility of those voices? At the click of a cursor, we can all now find someone who will agree with us, no matter how speculative our opinion may be.

All this made for an unpropitious context for the arrival of Covid-19 – an event which, even in more harmonious times, would surely have tested trust in public institutions. Conspiracy theories thrive on feelings of vulnerability, uncertainty and fear. The virus, invisible and deadly, delivered this in spades. Everyone found their life turned upside down, with little prospect of a speedy resolution. Governments imposed restrictions that were both unprecedented in scope and enforceable by law. To those isolated at home, with spare time plentiful, the online echo chamber was likely more seductive than ever. Let's not forget too that conspiracy thinking can deliver reassurance in difficult times. It provides a straightforward explanation for complex and frightening events, and with it a sense of control. It opens the door to a community of like-minded individuals. And it can allow people to feel that they have access to privileged information, thereby boosting their self-esteem. With Covid then, the conditions were right for conspiracy beliefs to move into the mainstream. And that may help explain why the link between conspiracy and marginalisation was less pronounced than in our 2016 research. Certainly, a lot of people in OCEANS who agreed with conspiracy beliefs also saw themselves as on the fringes of society. But many others didn't fall into this camp. Mistrust was now everywhere.

OCEANS II

'You must be unimaginably busy and apologies for the disturbance . . .'

By the time we published the OCEANS study, researchers at Oxford were already testing their Covid-19 vaccine on human volunteers. But what kind of reception, I wondered as I made my way across Port Meadow on my daily lockdown walk, would it eventually receive? A vaccination programme would rely on public trust – and that seemed to be in worryingly short supply. What could we do to counteract the levels of suspicion we'd discovered in OCEANS? How could we convince the millions of doubters that the pandemic was a genuine threat, to which a vaccine – and complementary public health measures – were an essential response?

As a first step, I needed to understand more about the kind of attitudes we'd discovered in OCEANS. I was also all too aware that, despite the importance of vaccination in overcoming Covid, I knew virtually nothing about the topic. Rather optimistically, I sent an email to Professor Sir Andrew Pollard, Director of the Oxford Vaccine Group, and Helen McShane, Professor of Vaccinology at the university. Amazingly, they replied. Even more surprisingly given the extraordinary pressure to produce a safe and effective Covid-19 vaccine in record time, they agreed to collaborate on what became OCEANS II. Joining the team too were Andrew Chadwick and Cristian Vaccari, political scientists at the Online Civic Culture Centre at Loughborough University. Unlike many, the dismaying picture painted by the first OCEANS project had not surprised them. On the contrary, its resonance with their own work had prompted them to get in touch with me. In 2018, Andrew and Cristian had discovered that remarkably large numbers of people are willing to report that they have shared exaggerated or made-up information on social media. (Over 40 per cent of people who shared news admitted to sharing inaccurate or false news, with 17.3 per cent sharing news they thought was made up when they shared it.)

OCEANS II was a two-part study: a survey of 5,100 UK adults, supplemented by in-depth interviews with people who held a range of views on vaccines. When we opened the survey on 27 September 2020, Covid-19 infections were on the rise again after a relatively benign summer and the relaxation of restrictions implemented in the spring. The situation was ominous. On 21 September, the government's Chief Scientific Officer had warned that by mid-October we could be seeing 50,000 new cases, and 200 deaths, every day. On 22 September, the prime minister announced further lockdown measures. Despite Boris Johnson's warning that the UK had 'reached a perilous turning point' and that 'unless we palpably make progress, we should assume that the restrictions that I have announced will remain in place for perhaps six months', OCEANS II showed that doubts about vaccination remained common. Just shy of 75 per cent of those we surveyed were enthusiastic about taking a vaccine, which by then was just a couple of months away from rollout. Around 15 per cent were strongly negative, asserting that they would never get vaccinated or would delay it for as long as they possibly could. The remaining 13 per cent sat on the fence – either they didn't know what they would do, or they would wait and see.

But these views didn't come out of nowhere. They had surprisingly little to do with the kind of demographic factors we'd seen in past work on conspiracy theories. Rather than being confined to the marginalised, mistrust was rather evenly distributed across the OCEANS II group. (Like the first OCEANS survey, the participants had been selected to be representative of age, gender, ethnicity, income, and region in the UK.) What principally explained conspiracy beliefs was how people felt about three key questions. The most important was the significance they attached to the *collective benefit* of getting themselves vaccinated. Those who were positive about the vaccine would say things like: 'So I think it's really selfish, almost, to think "Oh, I don't want to get it [the Covid-19 vaccine]" just because you think you'll be fine. It's about thinking about others and coming together sort of as like a community.' The vaccine hesitant, on the other hand, were more likely to emphasise personal choice: 'If I get it [the vaccine] then that's my choice. It's like if I smoke, that's my choice, if I want to shorten my life, because I know smoking will shorten my life. So it's just a personal choice thing.'

The second factor influencing attitudes was the speed with which the Covid-19 vaccines had been developed. For many, this was worthy of celebration: 'To get a vaccine ready in such a short time frankly is quite amazing and it shows how good our pharmaceutical industry is and I think it's something to be proud of.' For others, that rapidity was a red flag. Surely vaccines took longer to develop? And if the Covid vaccines were available so soon, risks must be inevitable:

'It's too short a time. I don't think there's anywhere enough data that they've got, and personally I think they may even, no definitely, they're using the general public as guinea pigs.'

'There was mass testing but it was over a shorter period of time than other vaccines had been. So, I think there could be so many side-effects in the long term that we don't know about. And we don't have time to find out about them . . . if I was to have children, I would be scared if it had an effect on them.'

That term 'guinea pigs' is one I heard a lot when I talked to vaccine-hesitant people. How, they wondered, could something so complex be devised and tested thoroughly in just a few months? Short cuts must have been taken. And that meant problems in the long run: 'no one knows the long-term effects. It's not been tested on anyone for that.' Trying to make sense of the speed with which the vaccine had been developed led some of our interviewees to even more pessimistic conclusions:

That was what people say, that it takes fifteen years before they can discover vaccines. But this one has taken only twelve months, or less than twelve months . . . This was so much quicker now, so I have to think, 'How is it going so much quicker?' I don't know. I didn't expect Covid-19 to happen before – is it manmade? When you plan something already, okay, let us plan Covid-19, plan for the medicine already. I don't know, maybe that is why it is quicker. I don't know.

The third key issue was the seriousness of the virus. 'It's no worse than the flu' was a claim we often heard from people sceptical about the vaccine. There was also a feeling that the authorities were cooking the epidemiological books: 'I still feel a lot of the figures are wrong because they seem to be putting things down to Covid where they're not all Covid. We know that, everybody knows it.' Those who were enthusiastic about the vaccine perceived the threat very differently: 'Obviously, surrounding areas have been bad, and the country as a whole has been a mess. A total mess. And it is serious because so many people are dying.'

And so they were. We published OCEANS II in December 2020. By the end of the month, the death toll in the UK had reached 72,000. In the US the figure was 375,000, and (according to the World Health Organization in May 2021) more than three million had died globally.

How people felt about these three questions really determined their attitude towards a Covid-19 vaccine: they were inextricably linked. Also important though were broader issues of trust. Those who were doubtful about the vaccine were also more likely to report negative views about doctors: 'They do not really care about me.' They were dubious about vaccine developers in general: 'They just want to make money.' They often said they'd had bad experiences with the NHS: 'Been put at the back of the queue for help'. They were open to conspiracy theories in general. And they displayed a nihilistic 'need for chaos' – an angry desire for society 'to be burned to the ground'. On the other hand, people who had enjoyed positive experiences with health professionals – 'My GP is polite and considerate'; 'Staff have gone out of their way to help me' – were much more amenable to a Covid-19 vaccine.

OCEANS II also reinforced the link between mistrust and low self-esteem. The more sceptical a person was of vaccination the worse they tended to feel about themselves in relation to other people. They were, they believed, lower on the social ladder – for example, in terms of their level of education, wealth and career. These people *felt* inferior. They felt vulnerable. And they were pretty doubtful that those at the top of the pile could be trusted to do the right thing by them.

OCEANS III

'It's so frustrating to see your loved ones blindly swallowing propaganda. I'm really scared about how many people will take this gene-altering vaccine because the government has lied and created all this fear.' (Julia)

How do we persuade people like Julia to take a vaccine that, despite all the scientific evidence to the contrary, they believe is unnecessary, ineffective and unsafe? Answering this question was the fundamental motivation for the OCEANS project, the destination to which I hoped the various studies would ultimately lead. And so, equipped with the insights from OCEANS II, we set out to discover whether we could craft messages that might shift these negative attitudes to Covid-19 vaccination. For example, if people don't appreciate the collective benefits of vaccination let's persuasively set out the case. Let's explain that the vaccines make it less likely that we'll pass on the virus, which means that by being vaccinated we're helping to protect each other: family, friends, neighbours and colleagues. Let's make the point that, although we might not be able to tell just by looking at them, some of the people we meet may be especially vulnerable to the effects of the virus. And by reducing the risk that we get severely ill, we can play our part in helping the country to bounce back as quickly as possible. We'll explain the seriousness of the virus and try to assuage the anxiety that the vaccine has been developed too quickly. That should help shift attitudes, shouldn't it?

To find out, in early February 2021 we surveyed nearly 15,000 UK adults, again carefully selected to be representative for age, gender, ethnicity, income and region. This was OCEANS III. First, we assessed vaccine hesitancy and were pleased to see that it had come down significantly – from 27 to 17 per cent – in the few months since OCEANS II. This was probably due at least in part to the fact that the vaccine was now very much with us. By the time we began recruiting participants, 4,609,740 first-dose vaccinations had been given in the UK and 460,625 second doses. The vaccine was rapidly becoming normalised. Follow-up interviews with people who'd taken part in OCEANS II captured some of this: 'I felt more positive about it because there were so many people that were having it done.' Developing too was a sense that vaccination might well be the only way to avoid further restrictions: 'If someone said to me today, you can have the vaccine today and you can . . . go where you want to go tomorrow, I would have it done now.' This was all good news, but of course we were especially interested in how those who *hadn't* changed their minds would respond to vaccine messaging. So, in addition to our original group of 15,000, we recruited a further 4,000 people who were still dubious about the vaccine.

In OCEANS III participants were randomly asked to read one of ten texts, each of which provided different information about the vaccine, prefaced by a simple statement taken from the NHS website: 'The coronavirus (Covid-19) vaccines are safe and effective, and give you the best protection against coronavirus. They have been approved by the independent Medicines and Healthcare products Regulatory Agency (MHRA).' After reading their allocated text, participants completed a questionnaire on their willingness to be vaccinated for Covid-19. The results of this largest ever study of Covid-19 vaccine messaging took us by surprise. As we've seen, OCEANS II suggested that beliefs about the collective benefits of vaccination were crucial. The extent to which people bought into that narrative seemed to determine their willingness to get a jab. But in fact the text that was most likely to change the minds of the 10 per cent who were strongly opposed to the vaccine emphasised not the collective but the *personal* benefits of vaccination. It pointed out that you can't be sure, even if you're relatively young and fit, that you won't get seriously ill or struggle with long-term Covid-related problems. Taking the vaccine would allow you to get on with your life without worrying about what the virus might have in store.

On reflection, this made sense. If you're vaccine hesitant you're probably more worried about the risk of taking the vaccine (which you likely think isn't ready to be offered to the public) than about catching the virus (the seriousness of which you suspect has been grossly exaggerated). And because you probably feel marginalised in society, the idea that you should get the vaccine to help other people won't cut it. Almost by definition, then, for this group messages that focus on the personal ramifications of Covid-19 are likely to be much more compelling. This isn't to say that the collective benefits angle can't work with the vaccine hesitant. Indeed, it may well have been a factor in the shift of attitudes we picked up among OCEANS III participants. But by the time we get to the relatively small hard core of sceptics, it's the personal risk versus personal benefit argument that carries most weight.

What about the view that the vaccines have emerged too quickly? It's an understandable fear: the vaccines did indeed arrive with unparalleled speed. Remember too that in the early stages of the pandemic the authorities played down expectations of a quick fix. So, in OCEANS III we included a text explaining that the speed of development reflects exceptional commitment, investment, and co-operation from scientists, governments, public health organizations, pharmaceutical companies – and tens of thousands of members of the public who volunteered to test the vaccines. And that any side effects don't suddenly appear months and years after vaccination. Because of the way vaccines work, quickly training the body's immune system to fight off a virus, any problems show up within a month and usually much sooner. Happily, this information did seem to reassure the vaccine hesitant.

Covid-19 will not disappear in the foreseeable future. We're all getting used to being called for regular vaccine boosters. Take-up of the Covid-19 vaccine in the UK has been high: by October 2022, 94 per cent of people had received at least one dose. But according to the UK Office for National Statistics, 20 per cent of those who have received a first dose are doubtful as to whether they'd take a booster. In the US, only around 70 per cent are fully vaccinated, with large variation across states (twenty states have yet to reach 60 per cent). So there remains a significant minority of people who aren't sure whether to get a jab – or who are resolved not to. Many of those sceptical individuals are young: OCEANS II, for example, found that younger adults were more likely to be vaccine hesitant and other surveys have produced similar results. And in a study led by my Oxford colleague Mina Fazel, we were alarmed to discover that only 50 per cent of 28,000 school children aged 9–18 were willing to take a Covid-19 vaccine. Thirty-seven per cent were undecided, and 13 per cent said they would opt out entirely. Behind these headlines, a couple of findings stood out. First, younger children were much more likely to have reservations about the vaccine. Only 35.7 per cent of nine-year-olds said they'd opt in; for thirteen-year-olds the figure was 51.3 per cent; and by the time we got to the seventeen-year-olds it had risen to 77.8 per cent. But if this seems like an argument for simply waiting for young people to mature, it doesn't really wash. (In any case, the fact that 80 per cent of seventeen-year-olds will take a vaccine isn't really a cause for celebration.) Because it wasn't simply the students' age that seemed to have a bearing on their attitudes. The young people who said they'd decline a vaccine, and those who were unsure, were more likely to come from deprived backgrounds. They spent longer on social media (and we've seen already in this chapter the role this may play in conspiracy thinking) and they believed they didn't really belong in their school community. They felt, in effect, marginalised. This was especially true for the adolescents in the 'opt out' group: they were more likely to report being bullied at school and it looked as if their levels of paranoia might be higher too.

All this means that the issue of vaccination messaging isn't going to diminish in importance any time soon. The interviews we conducted in OCEANS II highlighted the bewilderment and confusion caused by the pandemic, especially among those who were reluctant to get vaccinated: 'the entire pandemic has been very much like people not knowing what's going on'. People were desperate for information they could trust:

'When I'm trying to look at this stuff or people are sharing PDFs and white papers and yellow papers and all kinds of documentation from apparently this scientist or that scientist, or this lab or that lab, I have no idea who these people are, if they are credible, who funds them, are they invested in a company that would benefit from this decision or that decision? . . . We just don't know what is and what isn't real.'

'I think people are just generally worried about the fact that they do not know what they're putting in their body.'

Effective communication around Covid-19 vaccination will probably need to include some core elements – about safety and effectiveness, for instance. But information must also be crafted for specific audiences (such as young people). And when it's out there, we need to monitor and review its reception: getting it right may take several iterations. Perhaps most importantly of all, we must listen, understand concerns, and address them seriously. No message will be truly effective if the messenger has not earned trust. We need too to think hard about the medium we use to convey information. For instance, OCEANS II showed that 10 per cent of the UK population planned to use social media and messaging apps to discourage others from getting a Covid vaccine. In a sense, they were anti-vax activists. These people were also likely to get their information from online networks of friends or to avoid news altogether. How to reach them with authoritative information about the vaccine? For these groups, the best approach may be direct contact, either through local health services, workplaces, direct mail, community work, or even street advertising. Hearing from researchers, popular scientists, and the vaccine developers themselves – rather than, say, politicians – was also suggested by our OCEANS II group as a way of getting the message across to the vaccine hesitant.

* * *

OCEANS taught me a lot. Over the years I'd become used to the idea that paranoia is much more prevalent than most people had ever suspected. Now, I saw that conspiracy thinking too was commonplace. Mistrust had become mainstream. And if we hadn't realised it before, the pandemic proved just how much this matters. Combating Covid-19 has required a collective effort. It relies on us all to follow the guidance and, crucially, make the big decision to take a needle in the arm (several times). It depends, in other words, on *trust*: in our fellow citizens, in our leaders, in our scientific and clinical experts. OCEANS itself was a reminder of what can be achieved, even during really challenging circumstances, when we do work together. Without that cohesion, without that trust in one another, it's hard to get anything done. Worse, things begin to fall apart.

14.

Ticking time bombs

We began this book with talk of battles. Of time bombs, treachery and terror. Of trust in ruins.

In March 1983 Ronald Reagan, then president of the United States, travelled to Orlando, Florida to address the National Association of Evangelicals. Since the late 1970s, relations between the US and USSR had chilled and the arms race had intensified. As a result, pressure had grown for a freeze on nuclear weapons. For the West to adopt such a freeze unilaterally, Reagan argued, would be a dangerous error. In his view, the USSR was inherently aggressive: 'as good Marxist-Leninists, the Soviet leaders have openly and publicly declared that the only morality they recognise is that which will further their cause, which is world revolution. . . . I would agree to a freeze if only we could freeze the Soviets' global desires.' The Cold War, Reagan stressed, was much more than a struggle for dominance between political systems and nation states:

I urge you to speak out against those who would place the United States in a position of military and moral inferiority. . . . in your discussions of the nuclear freeze proposals, I urge you to beware the temptation of pride – the temptation of blithely declaring yourselves above it all and label both sides equally at fault, to ignore the facts of history and the aggressive impulses of an evil empire, to simply call the arms race a giant misunderstanding and thereby remove yourself from the struggle between right and wrong and good and evil.

For all Reagan's Manichean thunder in Florida, his views on the USSR were becoming rather more nuanced than it appeared. The Soviets' stockpiling of nuclear weapons, he came to believe, was primarily defensive: 'the more experience I had with the Soviet leaders and other heads of state who knew them, the more I came to realise that many Soviet officials feared us not only as adversaries but as potential aggressors who might hurl nuclear weapons at them in a first strike.' Reagan, long convinced of the horror of nuclear warfare, began to envisage a world free of such weapons. As part of this endeavour, two weeks after his 'evil empire' speech the president announced the Strategic Defense Initiative. SDI's aim, according to Reagan, was to devise a protective shield above the US and thus render nuclear weapons 'impotent and obsolete'.

In the White House, Reagan's views on nuclear deceleration were largely ignored. Secretary of State George Shultz observed to his aides: 'The president has noticed that no one pays any attention to him in spite of the fact that he speaks about this idea publicly and privately.' But in fact, Reagan was correct in his appraisal of the Soviet mindset. Fear and mistrust of the United States were endemic among the leadership (just as they were in Washington towards Moscow). SDI, for example, was widely interpreted as a hostile act. Like many in the West, Soviet scientists doubted its feasibility. But if SDI's stated aims were pie in the sky, the Soviets reasoned, surely the Americans knew that? And if they were pressing ahead regardless, that must mean they had some other end in mind. In the view of Alexander Nadiradze, a Soviet missile designer, SDI was actually cover for a plan to deploy nuclear weapons from space. As David Hoffman recounts in *The Dead Hand*, Nadiradze warned the Central Committee that the so-called missile defence plan was in fact an 'aggressive weapon that gives the USA a new possibility to deliver an instant nuclear strike against the Soviet Union'.

By then, of course, Reagan had found a new ally in his effort to build trust between the two superpowers. Mikhail Gorbachev became leader of the Soviet Union in March 1985. He sat down with Reagan for the first time that November in Geneva. Describing the meeting to Hoffman years later, Gorbachev explained: 'Somehow we extended a hand to each other, and started talking. He speaks English, I speak Russian, he understands nothing, and I understand nothing. But it seems there is a kind of dialogue being connected, a dialogue of the eyes.' At the end of the summit, when they shook hands again on a statement that a nuclear war could not be won and must never be fought, Gorbachev was astonished. 'Can you imagine what that meant? . . . It meant that everything we had been doing was an error.'

That first meeting produced no formal missile deal, but the relationship continued to develop. By the time of their fourth summit in Moscow in May 1988 a genuine rapport had been established. 'What we have decided to do,' commented Reagan, 'is talk to each other and not about each other, and that's working just fine.' Not everyone was convinced by this outbreak of harmony. US vice-president George H.W. Bush, for one, was sure that 'the Cold War is not over'. He was wrong. As we know, the thaw proved genuine. And the evil empire? No, Reagan told journalists in Moscow that May, 'You are talking about another time, another era.'

* * *

How do we overcome the toxic forces of fear and paranoia? How can we build trust, with regards both to the people we encounter in our day-to-day lives and society at large? Finding the answers to these questions is essential, I believe, for our personal wellbeing. Far too many of us are prey to unnecessary, futile fear. We feel embattled. We've lost the ability accurately to estimate danger and risk. And it warps our sense of the world around us. But the issue is also of critical importance if we are to mend our fractured and fractious communities, fissured by inequality, discrimination (a factor strongly linked with paranoia in our recent survey of ten thousand people in the UK), manufactured 'culture wars', and ubiquitous social media.

These are obviously hugely complex problems – which means there are no easy solutions. But we'll get nowhere until we start to take those problems seriously. We urgently need to talk about trust: its importance, the forces that undermine it, and the measures we can take to restore it. I reiterate: this is not about blindly accepting whatever we may be told by those in authority, nor about ignoring real threats to our personal safety. But we should strive to base our judgements on evidence rather than emotion – and insist that such evidence remain central to any meaningful definition of truth. (Writing about Russia's invasion of Ukraine, Luke Harding notes that 'the KGB regarded the concept of truth itself as a ludicrous bourgeois construct. In the Kremlin's relativistic universe, what mattered was the story you told.' In this, I would argue, the Kremlin is far from being an anomaly.)

Given the limitless data and numberless voices of the internet, and in a culture of fake news and deepfakes, such aspirations may seem fanciful. The media's penchant for hair-raising stories of danger, death and destruction – the 'if it bleeds, it leads' approach to news – doesn't help either. But it isn't impossible to restore trust. I have seen numerous patients jettison severe and long-standing paranoid thoughts. They've been able to move on from patterns of thinking, feeling and behaving that have caused them unhappiness for years. For most of us, nothing like such radical change is necessary. We could start by adopting the Russian proverb I mentioned in Chapter 1: *trust, but verify*. (The author Suzanne Massie taught the phrase to Reagan, who enjoyed using it during negotiations with the Soviets. In 2020 Trump's Secretary of State, Mike Pompeo, declared that when dealing with China one should 'distrust, but verify' – a sign of the times perhaps.)

The story of our changing approach to clinical paranoia is illustrative here. As we've seen, when I began my career as a psychology assistant in the early 1990s no one was much interested in the topic. Persecutory delusions were extremely common among patients diagnosed with schizophrenia, but they were regarded merely as a symptom. There was little interest in listening to patients describe their fears – indeed, some clinicians worried that doing so would only distress the patient further – let alone in the targeted treatment of delusions. They would vanish, it was hoped, as the antipsychotic medication kicked in. It's no wonder, then, that paranoia was poorly understood. Having made it this far in the book, you'll know just how much has been discovered since then about the experience of persecutory delusions, the impact they can have on patients' lives, and the factors that cause and fuel them. And in programmes like Feeling Safe, we've learned how we can treat paranoia, helping people to move from crippling fear back into the life they want to lead. Along the way, we've also realised that paranoia isn't confined to the approximately 1 per cent of people diagnosed with psychotic disorders. On the contrary: it is a fundamental part of human experience, almost as common as feelings of depression or anxiety. Everyone, after all, must constantly make decisions about whether to trust or mistrust. This everyday paranoia isn't really very different to the delusions; it is simply less severe and intense.

We've come a long way then in regard to understanding and treating paranoia. There is much more to be done, of course. The number one priority must be to improve patients' access to the most effective therapies. Right now, demand far outstrips supply. We talk a lot these days about the importance of mental health, but it is still the poor relation. The charity MQ, for example, estimates that between 2014 and 2017 spending on mental health research amounted to just over £9 per person affected by psychological conditions; the figure for cancer research alone was £228 per person affected. And in 2022 the NHS Confederation noted that: 'Today in the UK mental health problems account for 28 per cent of the burden of disease but only 13 per cent of NHS spending.' There are positive developments: an increase in clinical psychology training places in the UK, for instance. But it remains a situation in which we need to think creatively, exploiting the therapeutic power of technology.

Feeling Safe, for example, can transform patients' lives. It's the best treatment out there for persecutory delusions. Every year we train around one hundred therapists across the UK to deliver Feeling Safe. And the programme is beginning to make its way into other countries too. In the Netherlands, for instance, I've been collaborating with Eva Tolmeijer and David van den Berg at the Vrije Universiteit Amsterdam who are combining Feeling Safe with peer counselling – which involves coaching from people with lived experience of psychosis and persecutory delusions. But the six-month programme demands a lot of time from clinical psychologists, of whom there simply aren't enough. So, with the backing of the National Institute for Health and Care Research, we're developing a new guided online version of the treatment, Feeling Safer, that users can access whenever and wherever they like via a smartphone, computer or tablet. That online work can be supported by a range of mental health workers, with face-to-face sessions dedicated to the key task of accompanying patients into everyday situations (taking a bus, for example, or going shopping). Those sessions will give patients the chance to have someone alongside them as they practise the techniques they've learned online and to discover that, despite their fear, they are in fact safe. By 2027, we'll have designed and built the treatment, tested it in a randomised controlled trial with almost 500 patients, analysed its cost-effectiveness, and prepared the ground for a rollout across the NHS.

Meanwhile, gameChange is making its way into the world, both in the NHS and in the US. And we're developing entirely new virtual reality treatments too. Young people with psychosis are an especially vulnerable group. The distress and stigma often caused by psychotic experiences breed feelings of despair, defeat and worthlessness. Those feelings make the psychosis worse; the individual retreats from everyday life; fear and mistrust take root; and mental and physical health deteriorate still further. The earlier we can intervene, the better chance we have of forestalling this vicious cycle. So we're developing and trialling Phoenix, a VR therapy designed to build self-confidence in people aged 16–30. Phoenix is an automated treatment: a virtual therapist guides the user through a range of challenges, games and exercises, set on a virtual farm, in a lakeside forest and in a TV studio. What we're after here is to change the way users feel about themselves. Specifically, we want them to learn that they can make a difference; that they can handle activities that might seem scary or overwhelming; and that they can have fun. If we can do that, we should see a big upturn in users' self-confidence. A pilot study with twelve young people has produced exceptional results. By the time you read this, we'll know whether we have been able to replicate that success in a randomised controlled trial. And, I hope, be getting it out to the people who need it.

Early intervention to overcome fear underlies another VR project we're running right now. One of the surprise findings from our OCEANS research was the discovery that 10 per cent of instances of Covid-19 vaccine hesitancy could be explained by a fear of needles. For all the talk about duplicitous governments and untrustworthy medics, a far more basic form of fear was in play: injection anxiety. In fact, this anxiety was much more prevalent among the entire OCEANS cohort than we had predicted: a quarter of the group were affected. Besides vaccination, needles are one of the most fundamental tools of healthcare, crucial to the treatment of countless acute and chronic conditions ranging from diabetes and chemotherapy to asthma and dental problems. Indeed, according to the World Health Organization, around 25 billion injections are administered every year. And of course, they are essential in blood donation (one in ten people cite needle fears as a reason for not giving blood). When it comes to treating needle phobia, we don't lack quick and effective psychological therapies. These involve gradually exposing the patient to injection-related stimuli until their fears subside, and teaching the technique of applied tension to combat the fall in blood pressure that can lead to fainting. Three hours can be enough to produce incredible results, but very few people receive any treatment – again, largely because our mental health services are just not equipped to provide it. So we're developing an automated VR therapy aimed, because phobias normally start in childhood, at young people aged 13–18. And it's not just about conquering a fear of needles. Removing that feeling of dread will also, I think, help build trust in medicine and the professionals who provide it. (Worryingly, OCEANS suggested that a quarter of the population don't trust doctors.)

For all the progress on clinical paranoia, when it comes to wider mistrust – the kind that manifests itself in conspiracy theories, for instance – we're still pretty much at the start line. I don't think we can afford to wait much longer. The Covid-19 pandemic turned a very bright light on the problem. Trust was revealed as literally a matter of life and death. It functions as an invisible infrastructure analogous to the electricity grid or the water network. We all depend on it, though it can take a crisis for us to appreciate just how much. Other infrastructure, of course, also took a bashing during the pandemic. The telecommunications network, for example, was targeted by protesters during the early stages of the Covid-19 pandemic with dozens of attacks on mobile phone masts. The writer James Meek recalled:

> A friend, a BBC journalist, told me about a conversation he'd had with an acquaintance who began talking about the dangers of 5G and claimed that 'every time a new kind of electromagnetic energy is invented, it causes a new kind of disease, like the invention of radar caused Spanish flu.'
>
> 'But Spanish flu happened in 1918, and radar wasn't invented till the 1930s,' my friend said.
>
> 'You would say that, wouldn't you?' This was uttered without a trace of a smile.

As it happens, the BBC was also attacked – sometimes literally – for its coverage of the crisis. Perhaps unsurprisingly, OCEANS revealed that people who sought their news from the BBC were less likely to be receptive to conspiracy theories, both in general and in relation to Covid. The opposite was true for those who relied on friends and social media for their information.

Repairing our creaking infrastructure of trust is a huge task, for sure. There's little indication that the kind of factors now putting it under such severe pressure are going to relent any time soon. But if Cold Warriors like Reagan and Gorbachev could establish sufficient trust to work together, I believe there is hope for the rest of us.

Acknowledgements

Readers might get the impression from this book that I am a clinical psychologist in a hurry. Indeed I am: we urgently need to deliver positive change for patients attending mental health services. (My hair began to go grey in my early twenties.) None of the advances detailed in these pages could have happened without a wonderful research team. I would particularly like to thank: Felicity Waite, Louise Isham, Bryony Sheaves, Sinéad Lambe, Laina Rosebrock, Jason Freeman, Aitor Rovira, Rowan Diamond, Emma Černis, Nicola Collett, Rachel Lister, Jessica Bird, Ariane Beckley, Ginny Evans, Helen Beckwith, Katherine Pugh, Mar Rus-Calafell, Angus Antley, Andre Lages Miguel, Rupert Ward, Matt Bousfield, Josie McInerney, Sarah Reeve, Amy Langman, Eve Twivy, Emily Bold, Eleanor Chadwick, Ava Forkert, Poppy Brown, Lucy Jenner and Stephanie Rek. I apologise for the constant refrain of 'we have one or two things to do' – although of course we do.

One learns early to work with talented but also kind people. I am lucky to have amazing collaborators and colleagues. I would like to thank: Ly-Mee Yu, Aiden Loe, Thomas Kabir, Anke Ehlers, Richard Emsley, Ushma Galal, Mel Slater, David Kingdon, Angelica Ronald, Helen Startup, Anthony Morrison, Melissa Pyle, Rory Byrne, Liz Murphy, Charlotte Aynsworth, Belinda Lennox, Alan Stein, Mina Fazel, Matthew Broome,

Louise Johns, Richard Bentall, Emmanuelle Peters, Alison Brabban, Andrew Gumley, Robert Dudley, Alex Kenny, Matthias Schwannauer, Amy Hardy, Tom Ward, Russell Foster, Colin Espie, Allison Harvey, Andrew Molodynski, Eleanor Longden, Gary Willington, Kate Chapman, Kathy Greenwood, José Leal, Helen McShane, Andy Pollard, Andrew Chadwick, Michael Larkin, Ray Fitzpatrick, Bernhard Spanlang, Paul Harrison, Mark van der Gaag, David van den Berg, Eva Tolmeijer, Julia Sheffield, Aaron Brinen and Steve Hollon. The professional support teams in the departments of Psychiatry and Experimental Psychology at the University of Oxford and in Oxford Health NHS Foundation Trust have provided essential support; thank you to Bill Wells, Nick Raven, Justin Lowen, Moira Westwood, Philly White, Wayne Davies, Tracy Tompkins, Katie Breeze and Ruth Abrahams. Likewise, I am grateful to the secretariats at research funders such as the National Institute for Health and Care Research (NIHR), Wellcome Trust and the Medical Research Council (MRC), who always work hard to support the best science.

The early belief from Claire Hughes, my tutor (and later friend) at Cambridge, made all the difference. My work on paranoia began under the guidance of Philippa Garety, my PhD supervisor. Philippa is a pioneer in delusion research and treatment and it has been an honour to have had the chance to learn from her. I could not have been more fortunate in the 1990s to be a (very junior) member of an exceptional research group with Philippa, Elizabeth Kuipers, David Fowler, Paul Bebbington and Graham Dunn. I learnt so much from all of them (and enjoyed much laughter too). I miss Graham Dunn, the methodologist and statistician, who was always so kindhearted and insightful. His influence still pervades my work.

Other leaders in psychological treatment have provided further crucial mentorship. Chris Fairburn has been very generous in guidance. Aaron Beck was a great source of support, knowledge and insights. David Clark has been a considerable influence, showing how to develop and implement really effective psychological treatments.

Thank you to Luigi Bonomi, my agent at LBA, and Arabella Pike, Publishing Director at HarperCollins, who spotted I might have a story to tell. Arabella and Jo Thompson have provided sage advice on the text. The storytelling has been hugely improved by the skills of Jason Freeman, my brother. I am very grateful for his help.

Finally I wish to express my deep gratitude to the people who have shared their experiences of paranoia. It has been – and remains – a privilege to spend time talking with people who are often going through so much. The progress described in this book could not have happened without this dialogue, nor the diligence and courage shown by patients as they practise therapeutic techniques inside and outside the clinic room. I would like to thank the individuals who gave permission for me to use quotes from them in this book, including those who recounted their experiences in our BBC Radio 4 *History of Delusions* series. Names and details of patient experiences have been altered to protect anonymity and snatches of clinic conversations are fictionalised accounts.

Sources

Chapter 1

Bentall, R. P. (ed.) (1990). *Reconstructing Schizophrenia*. London: Routledge.

Boyd, T. and Gumley, A. (2007). 'An experiential perspective on persecutory paranoia: A grounded theory construction'. *Psychology and Psychotherapy: Theory, Research and Practice*, 80(1), 1–22.

Clark, D. M. (1999). 'Anxiety disorders: Why they persist and how to treat them'. *Behaviour Research and Therapy*, 37(1), S5–S27.

Freeman, D. (2007). 'Suspicious minds: The psychology of persecutory delusions'. *Clinical Psychology Review*, 27, 425–457.

Freeman, D. (2006). 'Delusions in the non-clinical population'. *Current Psychiatry Reports*, 8, 191–204.

Freeman, D., Emsley, R., Diamond, R., Collett, N., Bold, E., Chadwick, E., Isham, L., Bird, J., Edwards, D., Kingdon, D., Fitzpatrick, R., Kabir, T., Waite, F. and Oxford Cognitive Approaches to Psychosis Trial Study Group (2021). 'Comparison of a theoretically driven cognitive therapy (the Feeling Safe Programme) with befriending for the treatment of persistent persecutory delusions: a parallel, single-blind, randomised controlled trial'. *The Lancet Psychiatry*, 8, 696–707.

Freeman, D. and Garety, P. A. (1999). 'Worry, worry processes and dimensions of delusions: An exploratory investigation of a role for anxiety processes in the maintenance of delusional distress'. *Behavioural and Cognitive Psychotherapy*, 27, 47–62.

Freeman, D., Garety, P. A. and Kuipers, E. (2001). 'Persecutory delusions: Developing the understanding of belief maintenance and emotional distress'. *Psychological Medicine*, 31, 1293–1306.

Freeman, D., Garety, P., Kuipers, E., Fowler, D., Bebbington, P. E. and Dunn, G. (2007). 'Acting on persecutory delusions: The importance of safety seeking'. *Behaviour Research and Therapy*, 45, 89–99.

Freeman, D., Waite, F., Rosebrock, L., Petit, A., Causier, C., East, A., Jenner, L., Teale, A., Carr, L., Mulhall, S., Bold, E. and Lambe, S. (2022). 'Coronavirus conspiracy beliefs, mistrust, and compliance with government guidelines in England'. *Psychological Medicine*, 52, 251–263.

Greene, G. (1943). *The Ministry of Fear*. London: Vintage.

Kessler, R. C., Berglund, P., Demler, O., Jin, R., Merikangas, K. R. and Walters, E. E. (2005). 'Lifetime prevalence and age-of-onset distributions of DSM-IV disorders in the National Comorbidity Survey Replication'. *Archives of General Psychiatry*, 62(6), 593–602.

Kuipers, E., Fowler, D., Garety, P. A., Chisholm, D., Freeman, D., Dunn, G., Bebbington, P. E. and Hadley, C. (1998). 'The London–East Anglia Randomised Controlled Trial of Cognitive Behaviour Therapy for Psychosis III: Follow-up and economic evaluation at 18 months'. *British Journal of Psychiatry*, 173, 61–68.

Le Carré, J. (1974; 2018). *Tinker Tailor Soldier Spy*. Penguin Classics. Random House, UK.

Rutten, B. P. F., van Os, J., Dominguez, M. and Krabbendam, L. (2008). 'Epidemiology and social factors: Findings from The Netherlands mental health survey and incidence and incidence study (NEMESIS)'. In Freeman, D., Bentall, R. and Garety P. (eds). *Persecutory Delusions*. pp. 53–71. Oxford: Oxford University Press.

Salkovskis, P. M. (1991). 'The importance of behaviour in the maintenance of anxiety and panic: A cognitive account'. *Behavioural Psychotherapy*, 19, 6–19.

Salkovskis, P. M., Clark, D. M., Hackmann, A., Wells, A. and Gelder, M. G. (1999). 'An experimental investigation of the role of safety-seeking behaviours in the maintenance of panic disorder with agoraphobia'. *Behaviour Research and Therapy*, 37(6), 559–574.

Chapter 2

Bighelli, I., Salanti, G., Huhn, M., Schneider-Thomas, J., Krause, M., Reitmeir, C., Wallis, S., Schwermann, F., Pitschel-Walz, G., Barbui, C., Furukawa, T. and Leucht, S. (2018). 'Psychological interventions to reduce positive symptoms in schizophrenia: Systematic review and network meta-analysis'. *World Psychiatry*, 17, 316–329.

Bond, J., Kenny, A., Mesaric, A., Wilson, N., Pinfold, V., Kabir, T., Freeman, D., Waite, F., Larkin, M. and Robotham, D. J. (2022). 'A life more ordinary: A peer research method qualitative study of the Feeling Safe Programme for persecutory delusions'. *Psychology and Psychotherapy*, 95, 1108–1125.

Brabban, A., Byrne, R., Longden, E. and Morrison, A. P. (2017). 'The importance of human relationships, ethics and recovery-orientated values in the delivery of CBT for people with psychosis'. *Psychosis*, 9(2), 157–166.

Diamond, R., Bird, J., Waite, F., Bold, E., Chadwick, E., Collett, N. and Freeman, D. (2022). 'The physical activity profiles of patients with persecutory delusions'. *Mental Health and Physical Activity*, 23, 100462.

Fowler, D., Garety, P. and Kuipers, E. (1995). *Cognitive Behaviour Therapy for Psychosis: Theory and Practice*. John Wiley & Sons.

Freeman, D. (2011). 'Improving cognitive treatments for delusions'. *Schizophrenia Research*, 132, 135–139.

Freeman, D. (2016). 'Persecutory delusions: A cognitive perspective on understanding and treatment'. *The Lancet Psychiatry*, 3, 685–692.

Freeman, D., Bird, J., Loe, B., Kingdon, D., Startup, H., Clark, D., Ehlers, A., Černis, E., Wingham, G., Evans, N., Lister, R., Pugh, K., Cordwell, J. and Dunn, G. (2020). 'The Dunn Worry Questionnaire and the

Paranoia Worries Questionnaire: New Assessments of Worry'. *Psychological Medicine*, 50, 771–780.

Freeman, D., Bradley, J., Waite, F., Sheaves, B., DeWeever, N., Bourke, E., McInerney, J., Evans, N., Černis, E., Lister, R., Garety, P. and Dunn, G. (2016). 'Targeting recovery in persistent persecutory delusions: A proof of principle study of a new translational psychological treatment'. *Behavioural and Cognitive Psychotherapy*, 44, 539–552.

Freeman, D., Dunn, G., Startup, H., Pugh, K., Cordwell, J., Mander, H., Černis, E., Wingham, G., Shirvell, K. and Kingdon, D. (2015). 'Effects of cognitive behaviour therapy for worry on persecutory delusions in patients with psychosis (WIT): A parallel, single-blind, randomised controlled trial with a mediation analysis'. *The Lancet Psychiatry*, 2, 305–313.

Freeman, D., Emsley, R., Diamond, R., Collett, N., Bold, E., Chadwick, E., Isham, L., Bird, J., Edwards, D., Kingdon, D., Fitzpatrick, R., Kabir, T., Waite, F. and Oxford Cognitive Approaches to Psychosis Trial Study Group (2021). 'Comparison of a theoretically driven cognitive therapy (the Feeling Safe Programme) with befriending for the treatment of persistent persecutory delusions: A parallel, single-blind, randomised controlled trial'. *The Lancet Psychiatry*, 8, 696–707.

Freeman, D., Loe, B. S., Kingdon, D., Startup, H., Molodynski, A., Rosebrock, L., Brown, P., Sheaves, B., Waite, F. and Bird, J. C. (2021). 'The revised Green et al., Paranoid Thoughts Scale (R-GPTS): Psychometric properties, severity ranges, and clinical cut-offs'. *Psychological Medicine*, 51, 244–253.

Freeman, D., Rosebrock, L., Loe, B. S., Saidel, S., Freeman, J. and Waite, F. (2023). 'The Oxford Positive Self Scale: psychometric development of an assessment of cognitions associated with psychological well-being'. *Psychological Medicine*, pp. 1–9.

Freeman, D., Startup, H., Dunn, G., Wingham, G., Černis, E., Evans, N., Lister, R., Pugh, K., Cordwell, J. and Kingdon, D. (2014). 'Persecutory delusions and psychological well-being'. *Social Psychiatry and Psychiatric Epidemiology*, 49, 1045–1050.

Freeman, D., Taylor, K., Molodynski, A. and Waite, F. (2019). 'Treatable clinical intervention targets for patients with schizophrenia'. *Schizophrenia Research*, 211, 44–50.

Green, C., Freeman, D., Kuipers, E., Bebbington, P., Fowler, D., Dunn, G. and Garety, P. A. (2008). 'Measuring ideas of persecution and reference: The Green et al Paranoid Thought Scales (G-PTS)'. *Psychological Medicine*, 38, 101–111.

Gumley, A. and Schwannauer, M. (2006). *Staying Well After Psychosis: A Cognitive Interpersonal Approach to Recovery and Relapse Prevention*. John Wiley & Sons.

Haddock, G., Eisner, E., Boone, C., Davies, G., Coogan, C. and Barrowclough, C. (2014). 'An investigation of the implementation of NICE-recommended CBT interventions for people with schizophrenia'. *Journal of Mental Health*, 23(4), 162–165.

Kingdon, D. G. and Turkington, D. (1991). 'The use of cognitive behavior therapy with a normalizing rationale in schizophrenia. Preliminary report'. *Journal of Nervous and Mental Disease*, 179(4), 207–211.

Kuipers, E., Garety, P. A., Fowler, D., Dunn, G., Bebbington, P. E., Freeman, D. and Hadley, C. (1997). 'The London–East Anglia Randomised Controlled Trial of Cognitive Behaviour Therapy for Psychosis I: Effects of the treatment phase'. *British Journal of Psychiatry*, 171, 319–327.

McGlanaghy, E., Turner, D., Davis, G., Sharpe, H., Dougall, N., Morris, P., Prentice, W. and Hutton, P. (2021). 'A network meta-analysis of psychological interventions for schizophrenia and psychosis'. *Schizophrenia Research*, 228, 447–459.

Morrison, A. P. and Barratt, S. (2010). 'What are the components of CBT for psychosis? A Delphi study'. *Schizophrenia Bulletin*, 36(1), 136–142.

Morrison, A., Renton, J., Dunn, H., Williams, S. and Bentall, R. (2004). *Cognitive Therapy for Psychosis: A Formulation-Based Approach*. London: Routledge.

Peters, E., Crombie, T., Agbedjro, D., Johns, L. C., Stahl, D., Greenwood, K., Keen, N., Onwumere, J., Hunter, E., Smith, L.

and Kuipers, E. (2015). 'The long-term effectiveness of cognitive behavior therapy for psychosis within a routine psychological therapies service'. *Frontiers in Psychology*, 6, 1658.

Chapter 3

Beck, A. T. (1952). 'Successful outpatient psychotherapy of a chronic schizophrenic with a delusion based on borrowed guilt'. *Psychiatry*, 15(3), 305–312.

Beck, A. T. (1963). 'There is more on the surface than meets the eye'. Lecture presented in The Academy of Psychoanalysis, New York.

Bentall, R. P. (2003). *Madness Explained: Psychosis and Human Nature*. London: Penguin.

Bentall, R. P., Corcoran, R., Howard, R., Blackwood, N. and Kinderman, P. (2001). 'Persecutory delusions: A review and theoretical integration'. *Clinical Psychology Review*, 21(8), 1143–1192.

Berrios, G. E. (1996). *The History of Mental Symptoms: Descriptive Psychopathology Since the Nineteenth Century*. Cambridge: Cambridge University Press.

Bleuler, E. (1950). *Dementia Praecox or the Group of Schizophrenias*. New York: International Universities Press.

Braithwaite, R. (2008). 'Response to Freeman, D. et al (2008). Virtual reality study of paranoid thinking in the general population'. *British Journal of Psychiatry*, 192(4), 258–263.

Ebert, A. and Bär, K.-J. (2010). 'Emil Kraepelin: A pioneer of scientific understanding of psychiatry and psychopharmacology'. *Indian Journal of Psychiatry*, 52(2), 191–192.

Fowler, D., Freeman, D., Smith, B., Kuipers, E., Bebbington, P., Bashforth, H., Coker, S., Gracie, A., Dunn, G. and Garety, P. (2006). 'The Brief Core Schema Scales (BCSS): Psychometric properties and associations with paranoia and grandiosity in non-clinical and psychosis samples'. *Psychological Medicine*, 36, 749–759.

Freeman, D., Garety, P., Fowler, D., Kuipers, E., Dunn, G., Bebbington, P. and Hadley, C. (1998). 'The London–East Anglia randomised controlled trial of cognitive behaviour therapy for psychosis IV: Self-esteem and persecutory delusions'. *British Journal of Clinical Psychology*, 37, 415–430.

Freud, S. (2001). *The Standard Edition of the Complete Psychological Works*, Volume 14, *On the History of the Psycho-Analytic Movement, Papers on Metapsychology and Other Works*. London: Vintage.

Goode, E. (2000). 'A pragmatic man and his no-nonsense therapy'. *New York Times*, archive.nytimes.com/www.nytimes.com/library/national/science/health/011100hth-behavior-beck.html

Gregory, R. L. (2004). *The Oxford Companion to the Mind*. 2nd edn. Oxford: Oxford University Press.

Gunby, D., Carnegie, D. and Jackson, M. P. (2021). *The Works of John Webster*, Volume 4, *Sir Thomas Wyatt, Westward Ho, Northward Ho, The Fair Maid of the Inn*. Cambridge: Cambridge University Press.

Haslam, J. (1810). *Illustrations of Madness*. London.

Jaspers, K. (1963). *General Psychopathology*. Translated from German, 7th edn, by Hoenig, J. and Hamilton, M. W. Manchester: Manchester University Press.

Kraepelin, E. (1919). *Dementia Praecox and Paraphrenia*. Livingstone.

Leigh, D. (1955). 'John Haslam, M. D. – 1764–1844: Apothecary to Bethlem'. *Journal of the History of Medicine and Allied Sciences*, 10(1), 17–44.

Lester, D. (1975). 'The relationship between paranoid delusions and homosexuality'. *Archives of Sexual Behavior*, 4, 285–294.

Lewis, A. (1970). 'Paranoia and paranoid: A historical perspective'. *Psychological Medicine*, 1(1), 2–12.

Liberman, R. P., Teigen, J., Patterson, R. and Baker, V. (1973). 'Reducing delusional speech in chronic, paranoid schizophrenics'. *Journal of Applied Behavior Analysis*, 6(1), 57–64.

Mayer-Gross, W., Slater, E. and Roth, M. (1969). *Clinical Psychiatry*. London: Baillière, Tindall & Cassell.

McMonagle, T. and Sultana, A. (2000). 'Token economy for schizophrenia'. *Cochrane Database of Systematic Reviews*, 3, CD001473.

Murphy, P., Bentall, R., Freeman, D., O'Rourke, S. and Hutton, P. (2018). 'The paranoia as defence model of persecutory delusions: A systematic review and meta-analysis'. *The Lancet Psychiatry*, 5, 913–929.

Peters, E. R., Joseph, S. A. and Garety, P. A. (1999). 'Measurement of delusional ideation in the normal population: Introducing the PDI (Peters et al. Delusions Inventory)'. *Schizophrenia Bulletin*, 25(3), 553–576.

Porter, R. (1997). 'Bethlem/Bedlam: Methods of madness?' *History Today*, 47(10), 41–47.

Scull, A. (1999). 'Bethlem Demystified? Jonathan Andrews, Asa Briggs, Roy Porter, Penny Tucker and Keir Waddington, *The History of Bethlem*, London and New York, Routledge, 1997, pp. xiv, 752, illus., £150.00 (0-415-01773-4)'. *Medical History*, 43(2), 248–255.

Steinberg, H. and Himmerich, H. (2012). 'Johann Christian August Heinroth (1773–1843): The first professor of psychiatry as a psychotherapist'. *Journal of Religion and Health*, 51(2), 256–268.

Stockland, E. (2017). 'Patriotic natural history and sericulture in the French Enlightenment (1730–1780)'. *Archives of Natural History*, 44(1), 1–18.

Storr, A. (2001). *Freud: A Very Short Introduction*. Oxford: Oxford University Press.

Wincze, J. P., Leitenberg, H. and Agras, W. S. (1972). 'The effects of token reinforcement and feedback on the delusional verbal behavior of chronic paranoid schizophrenics'. *Journal of Applied Behavior Analysis*, 5, 247–262.

Chapter 4

Barlow, D. H. and Durand, V. M. (2005). *Abnormal Psychology: An Integrative Approach*. Belmont, CA: Wadsworth.

Bebbington, P. E., McBride, O., Steel, C., Kuipers, E., Radovanoviĉ, M., Brugha, T., Jenkins, R., Meltzer, H. I. and Freeman, D. (2013). 'The structure of paranoia in the general population'. *British Journal of Psychiatry*, 202(6), 419–427.

Elahi, A., Algorta, G. P., Varese, F., McIntyre, J. C. and Bentall, R. P. (2017). 'Do paranoid delusions exist on a continuum with subclinical paranoia? A multi-method taxometric study'. *Schizophrenia Research*, 190, 77–81.

Freeman, D. (2008). 'Studying and treating schizophrenia using virtual reality: A new paradigm'. *Schizophrenia Bulletin*, 34, 605–610.

Freeman, D., Freeman, J. and Garety, P. (2006). *Overcoming Paranoid and Suspicious Thoughts*. London: Robinson.

Freeman, D. and Garety, P. A. (2004). *Paranoia: The Psychology of Persecutory Delusions*. Hove: Psychology Press.

Freeman, D., Garety, P. A., Bebbington, P. E., Smith, B., Rollinson, R., Fowler, D., Kuipers, E., Ray, K. and Dunn, G. (2005). 'Psychological investigation of the structure of paranoia in a non-clinical population'. *British Journal of Psychiatry*, 186, 427–435.

Freeman, D., McManus, S., Brugha, T., Meltzer, H., Jenkins, R. and Bebbington, P. (2011). 'Concomitants of paranoia in the general population'. *Psychological Medicine*, 41, 923–936.

Freeman, D., Pugh, K., Antley, A., Slater, M., Bebbington, P., Gittins, M., Dunn, G., Kuipers, E., Fowler, D. and Garety, P. A. (2008). 'A virtual reality study of paranoid thinking in the general population'. *British Journal of Psychiatry*, 192, 258–263.

Freeman, D., Pugh, K., Vorontsova, N., Antley, A. and Slater, M. (2010). 'Testing the continuum of delusional beliefs: An experimental study using virtual reality'. *Journal of Abnormal Psychology*, 119, 83–92.

Freeman, D., Reeve, S., Robinson, A., Ehlers, A., Clark, D., Spanlang, B. and Slater, M. (2017). 'Virtual reality in the assessment, understanding, and treatment of mental health disorders'. *Psychological Medicine*, 47, 2393–2400.

Freeman, D., Slater, M., Bebbington, P. E., Garety, P. A., Kuipers, E., Fowler, D., Met, A., Read, C., Jordan, J. and Vinayagamoorthy, V. (2003). 'Can virtual reality be used to investigate persecutory ideation?' *Journal of Nervous and Mental Disease*, 191, 509–514.

Johns, L. C., Cannon, M., Singleton, N., Murray, R. M., Farrell, M., Brugha, T., Bebbington, P., Jenkins, R. and Meltzer, H. (2004). 'Prevalence and correlates of self-reported psychotic symptoms in the British population'. *British Journal of Psychiatry*, 185(4), 298–305.

Lanier, J. (2017). *Dawn of the New Everything: A Journey Through Virtual Reality*. London: Bodley Head.

Marmoy, C. F. A. (1958). 'The "Auto-Icon" of Jeremy Bentham at University College, London'. *Medical History*, 2(2), 77–86.

McManus, S., Bebbington, P., Jenkins, R. and Brugha, T., eds. (2016). *Mental Health and Wellbeing in England: Adult Psychiatric Morbidity Survey 2014*. Leeds: NHS Digital.

Olfson, M., Lewis-Fernández, R., Feder, A., Gameroff, M., Pilowsky, D. and Fuentes, M. (2002). 'Psychotic symptoms in an urban general medicine practice'. *American Journal of Psychiatry*, 59, 1412–1419.

Rheingold, H. (1991). *Virtual Reality*. New York: Simon & Schuster.

Sanchez-Vives, M. V. and Slater, M. (2005). 'From presence to consciousness through virtual reality'. *Nature Reviews Neuroscience*, 6(4), 332–339.

Slater, M. (2009). 'Place illusion and plausibility can lead to realistic behaviour in immersive virtual environments'. *Philosophical Transactions of the Royal Society B: Biological Sciences*, 364(1535), 3549–3557.

Slater, M., Rovira, A., Southern, R., Swapp, D., Zhang, J. J., Campbell, C. and Levine, M. (2013). 'Bystander responses to a violent incident in an immersive virtual environment'. *PLoS One*, 8(1), e52766.

Sutherland, I. A. (1968). 'Head-mounted three dimensional display'. *Proceedings of the Joint Computer Conference*, 33, 757–764.

Tien, A. Y. and Eaton, W. W. (1992). 'Psychopathologic precursors and sociodemographic risk factors for the schizophrenia syndrome'. *Archives of General Psychiatry*, 49(1), 37–46.

World Health Organization (2002). 'Schizophrenia', www.who.int/news-room/fact-sheets/detail/schizophrenia

Chapter 5

All Party Parliamentary Group for UN Women (2021). 'Prevalence and reporting of sexual harassment in UK public spaces'. APPG for UN Women, www.unwomenuk.org/site/wp-content/uploads/2021/03/APPG-UN-Women-Sexual-Harassment-Report_Updated.pdf

Alsawy, S., Wood, L., Taylor, P. J. and Morrison, A. P. (2015). 'Psychotic experiences and PTSD: Exploring associations in a population survey'. *Psychological Medicine*, 45(13), 2849–2859.

Armitage, R. (2021). 'Bullying in children: Impact on child health'. *BMJ Paediatrics Open*, 5(1), E000939.

Barker, M. (2000). 'Bullying: Schoolmates "told me to die" in online posts'. BBC News, www.bbc.co.uk/news/uk-wales-55133454

Bentall, R. P., Wickham, S., Shevlin, M. and Varese, F. (2012). 'Do specific early-life adversities lead to specific symptoms of psychosis? A study from the 2007 Adult Psychiatric Morbidity Survey'. *Schizophrenia Bulletin*, 38(1), 734–740.

Bird, J. C., Evans, R., Waite, F., Loe, B. S. and Freeman, D. (2019). 'Adolescent paranoia: Prevalence, structure, and causal mechanisms'. *Schizophrenia Bulletin*, 45, 1134–1142.

Bird, J. C., Fergusson, E. C., Kirkham, M., Shearn, C., Teale, A. L., Carr, L., Stratford, H. J., James, A. C., Waite, F. and Freeman, D. (2021). 'Paranoia in patients attending child and adolescent mental health services'. *Australian and New Zealand Journal of Psychiatry*, 55, 1166–1177.

Bird, J., Freeman, D. and Waite, F. (2022). 'The journey of adolescent paranoia: A qualitative study with patients attending child and adolescent mental health services'. *Psychology and Psychotherapy*, 95(2), 508–524.

Campbell, M. L. and Morrison, A. P. (2007). 'The relationship between bullying, psychotic-like experiences and appraisals in 14–16-year olds'. *Behaviour Research and Therapy*, 45(7), 1579–1591.

Catone, G., Marwaha, S., Kuipers, E., Lennox, B., Freeman, D.,

Bebbington, P. and Broome, M. (2015). 'Bullying victimisation and risk of psychotic phenomena: Analyses of British national survey data'. *The Lancet Psychiatry*, 2, 618–624.

Černis, E., Evans, R., Ehlers, A. and Freeman, D. (2021). 'Dissociation in relation to other mental health conditions: An exploration using network analysis'. *Journal of Psychiatric Research*, 136, 460–467.

Cosslett, R. L. (2018). '"I feel I might die any waking moment": can I escape the grip of PTSD?' *Guardian*, www.theguardian.com/society/2018/oct/20/feel-might-die-post-traumatic-stress-disorder-ptsd

Ehlers, A. and Clark, D. M. (2000). 'A cognitive model of posttraumatic stress disorder'. *Behaviour Research and Therapy*, 38(4), 319–345.

Freeman, D. and Fowler, D. (2009). 'Routes to psychotic symptoms: Trauma, anxiety and psychosis-like experiences'. *Psychiatry Research*, 169, 107–112.

Freeman, D., McManus, S., Brugha, T., Meltzer, H., Jenkins, R. and Bebbington, P. (2011). 'Concomitants of paranoia in the general population'. *Psychological Medicine*, 41, 923–936.

Freeman, D., Thompson, C., Vorontsova, N., Dunn, G., Carter, L-A., Garety, P., Kuipers, E., Slater, M., Antley, A., Glucksman, E. and Ehlers, A. (2013). 'Paranoia and post-traumatic stress disorder in the months after a physical assault: A longitudinal study examining shared and differential predictors'. *Psychological Medicine*, 43, 2673–2684.

Hardy, A., O'Driscoll, C., Steel, C., Van Der Gaag, M. and Van Den Berg, D. (2021). 'A network analysis of post-traumatic stress and psychosis symptoms'. *Psychological Medicine*, 51(14), 2485–2492.

Kasperkevic, J. (2014). 'Accounts of bullying at work: "it's subtle, political and leaves you unsure"'. *Guardian*, www.theguardian.com/money/us-money-blog/2014/jul/06/bullying-at-work-political-experiences-bullies-solutions

McManus, S., Bebbington, P. E., Jenkins, R. and Brugha, T. (2016).

Mental Health and Wellbeing in England: The Adult Psychiatric Morbidity Survey 2014. Leeds: NHS Digital.

Modecki, K. L., Minchin, J., Harbaugh, A. G., Guerra, N. G. and Runions, K. C. (2014). 'Bullying prevalence across contexts: A meta-analysis measuring cyber and traditional bullying'. *Journal of Adolescent Health*, 55(5), 602–611.

Morrison, A. P., Frame, L. and Larkin, W. (2003). 'Relationships between trauma and psychosis: A review and integration'. *British Journal of Clinical Psychology*, 42(Pt 4), 331–353.

Nielsen, M. B., Matthiesen, S. B. and Einarsen, S. (2010). 'The impact of methodological moderators on prevalence rates of workplace bullying: A meta-analysis'. *Journal of Occupational and Organizational Psychology*, 83, 955–979.

Office for National Statistics (2022). 'The nature of violent crime in England and Wales: Year ending March 2022', www.ons.gov.uk/peoplepopulation and community/crimeandjustice/articles/thenatureofviolentcrimeinenglandandwales/yearendingmarch2022

Shakoor, S., McGuire, P., Cardno, A. G., Freeman, D., Plomin, R. and Ronald, A. (2015). 'A shared genetic propensity underlies experiences of bullying victimization in late childhood and self-rated paranoid thinking in adolescence'. *Schizophrenia Bulletin*, 41(3), 754–763.

Smith, S. G., Zhang, X., Basile, K. C., Merrick, M. C., Wang, J., Kresnow, M.-J. and Chen, J. (2018). *National Intimate Partner and Sexual Violence Survey: 2015 Data Brief – Updated Release*. Atlanta, GA: National Center for Injury Prevention and Control, www.cdc.gov/violenceprevention/pdf/2015data-brief508.pdf

UNESCO (2017). *School Violence and Bullying: Global status report*. Paris: UNESCO.

van der Vleugel, B. M., Libedinsky, I., de Bont, P. A., de Roos, C., van Minnen, A., de Jongh, A., van der Gaag, M. and van den Berg, D. (2020). 'Changes in posttraumatic cognitions mediate the effects of trauma-focused therapy on paranoia'. *Schizophrenia Bulletin Open*, 1(1), sgaa036.

Chapter 6

Baker, C. (2023). 'Obesity statistics'. Research Briefing 3336. UK Parliament, commonslibrary.parliament.uk/research-briefings/sn03336/

Bowlby, J. (1967). Foreword to Mary D. Salter Ainsworth, *Infancy in Uganda*. Baltimore: Johns Hopkins.

Brenan, M. (2022). 'Record high 56% in U.S. perceive local crime has increased'. Gallup, news.gallup.com/poll/404048/record-high-perceive-local-crime-increased.aspx

Brown, P., Waite, F. and Freeman, D. (2020). 'Parenting behaviour and paranoia: A network analysis and results from the National Comorbidity Survey-Adolescents (NCS-A)'. *Social Psychiatry and Psychiatric Epidemiology*, 56, 593–604.

Freeman, D. and Bentall, R. (2017). 'The concomitants of conspiracy concerns'. *Social Psychiatry and Psychiatric Epidemiology*, 52, 595–604.

Fusar-Poli, P. et al. (2022). 'The lived experience of psychosis: A bottom-up review co-written by experts by experience and academics'. *World Psychiatry*, 21(2), 168–188.

Gerull, F. and Rapee, R. (2002). 'Mother knows best: Effects of maternal modelling on the acquisition of fear and avoidance behaviour in toddlers'. *Behaviour Research and Therapy*, 40, 279–287.

Jaspers, K. (1997). *General Psychopathology*. Baltimore and London: Johns Hopkins University Press.

Laneri, R. (2017). 'I went to jail for leaving my baby outside a restaurant'. *New York Post*, nypost.com/2017/11/25/i-went-to-jail-for-leaving-my-baby-outside-a-restaurant/

Maudsley, H. (1873). *Body and Mind*. London: Macmillan.

Maudsley, H. (1912; 1988). 'Autobiography'. *British Journal of Psychiatry*, 153, 736–740.

McCann, T. V., Lubman, D. I. and Clark, E. (2011). 'First-time primary caregivers' experience of caring for young adults with first-episode psychosis'. *Schizophrenia Bulletin*, 37(2), 381–388.

Office for National Statistics (2017). 'People greatly overestimate their likelihood of being robbed', www.ons.gov.uk/peoplepopulation-andcommunity/crimeandjustice/articles/peoplegreatlyoverestimatetheirlikelihoodofbeingrobbed/2017-09-07

Onwumere, J., Learmonth, S. and Kuipers, E. (2016). 'Caring for a relative with delusional beliefs: A qualitative exploration'. *Journal of Psychiatric and Mental Health Nursing*, 23(3–4), 145–155.

Pantelidou, M. and Demetriades, A. K. (2014). 'The enigmatic figure of Dr Henry Maudsley (1835–1918)'. *Journal of Medical Biography*, 22(3), 180–188.

Plomin, R., DeFries, J. C. and McClearn, G. E. (2008). *Behavioral Genetics*. New York: Worth Publishers.

Ronald, A. (2015). 'Recent quantitative genetic research on psychotic experiences: new approaches to old questions'. *Current Opinion in Behavioral Sciences*, 2, 81–88.

Roser, M. and Ortiz-Ospina, E. (2016). *Trust*. Our World in Data, ourworldindata.org/trust

Savage, G. H. (1918). 'Henry Maudsley, M.D., F.R.C.P.Lond., Ll.D.Edin. (Hon.)'. *Journal of Mental Science*, 64.265, 116–129.

Sieradzka, D., Power, R., Freeman, D., Cardno, A., Dudbridge, F. and Ronald, A. (2015). 'Heritability of individual psychotic experiences captured by common genetic variants in a community sample of adolescents'. *Behavior Genetics*, 45, 493–502.

Sieradzka, D., Power, R. A., Freeman, D., Cardno, A. G., McGuire, P., Plomin, R., Meaburn, E. L., Dudbridge, F. and Ronald, A. (2014). 'Are genetic risk factors for psychosis also associated with dimension-specific psychotic experiences in adolescence?' *PLoS One*, 9(4), e94398.

Smith, L., Onwumere, J., Craig, T., McManus, S., Bebbington, P. and Kuipers, E. (2014). 'Mental and physical illness in caregivers: Results from an English national survey sample'. *British Journal of Psychiatry*, 205(3), 197–203.

Stanley, A. P. (1844). 'The life and correspondence of Thomas Arnold, D.D.: Late head master of Rugby School and regius professor of modern history in the University of Oxford'. London: B. Fellowes.

Sündermann, O., Onwumere, J., Bebbington, P. and Kuipers, E. (2013). 'Social networks and support in early psychosis: Potential mechanisms'. *Epidemiology and Psychiatric Sciences*, 22(2), 147–150.

Sündermann, O., Onwumere, J., Kane, F., Morgan, C. and Kuipers, E. (2014). 'Social networks and support in first-episode psychosis: Exploring the role of loneliness and anxiety'. *Social Psychiatry and Psychiatric Epidemiology*, 49(3), 359–366.

Taylor, M. J., Freeman, D., Lundström, S., Larsson, H. and Ronald, A. (2022). 'Heritability of psychotic experiences in adolescents and interaction with environmental risk'. *JAMA Psychiatry*, 79(9), 889–897.

Weale, S. (2021). 'UK children not allowed to play outside until two years older than parents' generation'. *Guardian*, www.theguardian.com/society/2021/apr/20/gradual-lockdown-of-uk-children-as-age-for-solo-outdoor-play-rises

Zavos, H. M. S., Freeman, D., Haworth, C. M. A., McGuire, P., Plomin, R., Cardno, A. G. and Ronald, A. (2014). 'Consistent etiology of severe, frequent psychotic experiences and milder, less frequent manifestations: A twin study of specific psychotic experiences in adolescence'. *JAMA Psychiatry*, 71, 1049–1057.

Chapter 7

Adjaye-Gbewonyo, D., Ng, A. E. and Black, L. I. (2022). 'Sleep difficulties in adults: United States, 2020', Hyattsville, MD: National Center for Health Statistics: www.cdc.gov/nchs/data/databriefs/db436.pdf

Bradley, J., Freeman, D., Chadwick, E., Harvey, A. G., Mullins, B., Johns, L., Sheaves, B., Lennox, B., Broome, M. and Waite, F. (2018). 'Treating sleep problems in young people at ultra-high risk of psychosis: A feasibility case series'. *Behavioural and Cognitive Psychotherapy*, 46, 276–291.

Espie, C. (2021). *Overcoming Insomnia: A Self-Help Guide Using Cognitive Behavioural Techniques.* 2nd edn. London: Robinson.

Fitzgerald, F. Scott (1945; 2018). *The Crack-Up*. Richmond, VA: Alma.

Foster, R. (2022). *Life Time: The New Science of the Body Clock, and How It Can Revolutionize Your Sleep and Health*. London: Penguin.

Freeman, D., Brugha, T., Meltzer, H., Jenkins, R., Stahl, D. and Bebbington, P. (2010). 'Persecutory ideation and insomnia: findings from the second British National Survey of Psychiatric Morbidity'. *Journal of Psychiatric Research*, 44, 1021–1026.

Freeman, D., Pugh, K., Vorontsova, N. and Southgate, L. (2009). 'Insomnia and paranoia'. *Schizophrenia Research*, 108, 280–284.

Freeman, D., Stahl, D., McManus, S., Meltzer, H., Brugha, T., Wiles, N. and Bebbington, P. (2012). 'Insomnia, worry, anxiety and depression as predictors of the occurrence and persistence of paranoid thinking'. *Social Psychiatry and Psychiatric Epidemiology*, 47, 1195–1203.

Freeman, D., Sheaves, B., Goodwin, G., Yu, L-M., Nickless, A., Harrison, P., Emsley, R., Luik, A., Foster, R., Wadekar, V., Hinds, C., Gumley, A., Jones, R., Lightman, S., Jones, S., Bentall, R., Kinderman, P., Rowse, G., Brugha, T., Blagrove, M., Gregory, A., Fleming, L., Walklet, E., Glazebrook, C., Davies, E., Hollis, C., Haddock, G., John, B., Coulson, M., Fowler, D., Pugh, K., Cape, J., Mosely, P., Brown, G., Hughes, C., Obonsawin, M., Coker, S., Watkins, E., Schwannauer, M., MacMahon, K., Siriwardena, A. and Espie, C. (2017). 'The effects of improving sleep on mental health (OASIS): A randomised controlled trial with mediation analysis'. *The Lancet Psychiatry*, 4, 749–758.

Freeman, D., Sheaves, B., Waite, F., Harvey, A. and Harrison, P. (2020). 'Sleep disturbance and psychiatric disorders: The non-specific as essential in understanding and treating mental ill health'. *Lancet Psychiatry*, 7, 628–637.

Freeman, D., Waite, F., Startup, H., Myers, E., Lister, E., McInerney, J., Harvey, A., Geddes, J., Zaiwalla, Z., Luengo-Fernandez, R., Foster, R., Clifton, L. and Yu, L.-M. (2015). 'Efficacy of cognitive behavioural therapy for sleep improvement in patients with persistent delusions and hallucinations (BEST): A prospective, assessor-blind, randomised controlled pilot study'. *The Lancet Psychiatry*, 2, 975–983.

Hennig, T. and Lincoln,T. (2018). 'Sleeping paranoia away? An actigraphy and experience-sampling study with adolescents'. *Child Psychiatry and Human Development*, 49(1), 63–72.

Katz, S. E. and Landis, C. (1935). 'Psychologic and physiologic phenomena during a prolonged vigil'. *Archives of Neurology and Psychiatry*, 34(2), 307–317.

Koyanagi, A. and Stickley, A. (2015). 'The association between sleep problems and psychotic symptoms in the general population: A global perspective'. *Sleep*, 38(12), 1875–1885.

Reeve, S., Emsley, R., Sheaves, B. and Freeman, D. (2018). 'Disrupting sleep: The effects of sleep loss on psychotic experiences tested in an experimental study with mediation analysis'. *Schizophrenia Bulletin*, 44, 662–671.

Reeve, S., Sheaves, B. and Freeman, D. (2019). 'Sleep disorders in early psychosis: Incidence, severity, and association with clinical symptoms'. *Schizophrenia Bulletin*, 45, 287–295.

Reeve, S., Sheaves, B. and Freeman, D. (2021) 'Excessive sleepiness in patients with psychosis: An initial investigation'. *PLoS One* 16,(1), e0245301.

Rehman, A., Waite, F., Sheaves, B., Biello, S., Freeman, D. and Gumley, A. (2017). 'Clinician perceptions of sleep problems and their treatment in patients with non-affective psychosis'. *Psychosis*, 9, 129–139.

Sheaves, B., Freeman, D., Isham, L., McInerney, J., Nickless, A., Yu, L.-M., Rek, S., Bradley, J., Reeve, S., Attard, C., Espie, C. A., Foster, R., Wirz-Justice, A., Chadwick, E. and Barrera, A. (2018). 'Stabilising sleep for patients admitted at acute crisis to a psychiatric hospital (OWLS): An assessor-blind pilot randomised controlled trial'. *Psychological Medicine*, 48, 1694–1704.

Sheaves, B., Holmes, E. A., Rek, S., Taylor, K. M., Nickless, A., Waite, F., Germain, A., Espie, C. A., Harrison, P. J., Foster, R. and Freeman, D. (2019). 'Cognitive behavioural therapy for nightmares for patients with persecutory delusions (Nites): An assessor-blind, pilot randomized controlled trial'. *Canadian Journal of Psychiatry*, 64, 686–696.

Sheaves, B., Isham, L., Bradley, J., Espie, C., Barrera, A., Waite, F., Harvey, A., Attard, C. and Freeman, D. (2018). 'Adapted CBT to stabilize sleep on psychiatric wards'. *Behavioural and Cognitive Psychotherapy*, 46, 661–675.

Tandon, R., Lenderking, W. R., Weiss, C., Shalhoub, H., Dias Barbosa, C., Chen, J., Greene, M., Meehan, S. R., Duvold, L. B., Arango, C., Agid, O. and Castle, D. (2020). 'The impact on functioning of second-generation antipsychotic medication side effects for patients with schizophrenia: A worldwide, cross-sectional, web-based survey'. *Annals of General Psychiatry*, 19(1), 42.

Taylor, M., Gregory, A., Freeman, D. and Ronald, A. (2015). 'Do sleep disturbances and psychotic experiences in adolescence share genetic and environmental influences?' *Journal of Abnormal Psychology*, 124, 674–684.

Waite, F., Bradley, J., Chadwick, E., Reeve, S., Bird, J. and Freeman, D. (2018). 'The experience of sleep problems and their treatment in young people at ultra-high risk of psychosis: a thematic analysis'. *Frontiers in Psychiatry*, 9, 375.

Waite, F., Černis, E., Kabir, T., Iredale, E., Johns, L., Maughan, D., Diamond, R., Seddon, R., Williams, N., SleepWell Lived Experience Advisory Group, Yu, L.-M. and Freeman, D. (2023). 'A targeted psychological treatment for sleep problems in young people at ultra-high risk of psychosis in England (SleepWell): A parallel group, single-blind, randomised controlled feasibility trial'. *Lancet Psychiatry*, 10(9), 706–708.

Waite, F., Evans, N., Myers, E., Startup, H., Lister, R., Harvey, A. G. and Freeman, D. (2016). 'The patient experience of sleep problems and their treatment in the context of current delusions and hallucinations'. *Psychology and Psychotherapy: Theory, Research and Practice*, 89, 181–193.

Waite, F., Kabir, T., Johns, L., Mollison, J., Tsiachristas, A., Petit, A., Černis, E., Maughan, D. and Freeman, D. (2020). 'Treating sleep problems in young people at ultra-high risk of psychosis: Study protocol for a single-blind parallel group randomised controlled feasibility trial (SleepWell)'. *BMJ Open*, 10:e045235.

Waite, F., Myers, E., Harvey, A., Espie, C., Startup, H., Sheaves, B. and Freeman, D. (2016). 'Treating sleep problems in patients with schizophrenia'. *Behavioural and Cognitive Psychotherapy*, 44, 273–287.

Wulff, K., Dijk, D.-J., Middleton, B., Foster, R. G. and Joyce, E. M. (2012). 'Sleep and circadian rhythm disruption in schizophrenia'. *British Journal of Psychiatry*, 200, 308–316.

Youngstedt, S. D. et al. (2016). 'Has adult sleep duration declined over the last 50+ years?' *Sleep Medicine Reviews*, 28, 65–81.

Chapter 8

Atherton, S., Antley, A., Evans, N., Černis, E., Lister, R., Dunn, G., Slater, M. and Freeman, D. (2016). 'Self-confidence and paranoia: An experimental study using an immersive virtual reality social situation'. *Behavioural and Cognitive Psychotherapy*, 44, 56–64.

Bentall, R. P., Rowse, G., Shryane, N., Kinderman, P., Howard, R., Blackwood, N., Moore, R. and Corcoran, R. (2009). 'The cognitive and affective structure of paranoid delusions: A transdiagnostic investigation of patients with schizophrenia spectrum disorders and depression'. *Archives of General Psychiatry*, 66, 236–247.

Blaker, N. M., Rompa, I., Dessing, I. H., Vriend, A. F., Herschberg, C. and Van Vugt, M. (2013). 'The height leadership advantage in men and women: Testing evolutionary psychology predictions about the perceptions of tall leaders'. *Group Processes and Intergroup Relations*, 16(1), 17–27.

Bird, J. C., Waite, F., Rowsell, E., Fergusson, E. C. and Freeman, D. (2017). 'Cognitive, affective, and social factors maintaining paranoia in adolescents with mental health problems: A longitudinal study'. *Psychiatry Research*, 257, 34–39.

Bolier, L., Haverman, M., Westerhof, G. J. et al. (2013). 'Positive psychology interventions: A meta-analysis of randomized controlled studies'. *BMC Public Health*, 13, 119.

Brontë, E. (1847; 2003). *Wuthering Heights*. London: Penguin.

Brown, P., Waite, F., Rovira, A., Nickless, A. and Freeman, D. (2020). 'Virtual reality clinical-experimental tests of compassion treatment techniques to reduce paranoia'. *Scientific Reports*, 10, 8547.

Carr, A., Cullen, K., Keeney, C., Canning, C., Mooney, O., Chinseallaigh, E. and O'Dowd, A. (2021). 'Effectiveness of positive psychology interventions: A systematic review and meta-analysis'. *Journal of Positive Psychology*, 16(6), 749–769.

Forkert, A., Brown, P., Freeman, D. and Waite, F. (2022). 'A compassionate imagery intervention for patients with persecutory delusions'. *Behavioural and Cognitive Psychotherapy*, 50, 15–27.

Fowler, D., Freeman, D., Smith, B., Kuipers, E., Bebbington, P., Bashforth, H., Coker, S., Gracie, A., Dunn, G. and Garety, P. (2006). 'The Brief Core Schema Scales (BCSS): Psychometric properties and associations with paranoia and grandiosity in non-clinical and psychosis samples'. *Psychological Medicine*, 36, 749–759.

Freeman, D., Bold, E., Chadwick, E., Taylor, K., Collett, N., Diamond, R., Černis, E., Bird, J., Isham, L., Forkert, A., Carr, L., Causiera, C. and Waite, F. (2019). 'Suicidal ideation and behaviour in patients with persecutory delusions: Prevalence, symptom associations, and psychological correlates'. *Comprehensive Psychiatry*, 93, 41–47.

Freeman, D., Evans, N., Lister, R., Antley, A., Dunn, G. and Slater, M. (2014). 'Height, social comparison, and paranoia: An immersive virtual reality experimental study'. *Psychiatry Research*, 30, 348–352.

Freeman, D., Garety, P., Fowler, D., Kuipers, E., Dunn, G., Bebbington, P. and Hadley, C. (1998). 'The London–East Anglia randomised controlled trial of cognitive behaviour therapy for psychosis IV: Self-esteem and persecutory delusions'. *British Journal of Clinical Psychology*, 37, 415–430.

Freeman, D., Pugh, K., Dunn, G., Evans, N., Sheaves, B., Waite, F., Černis, E., Lister, R. and Fowler, D. (2014). 'An early Phase II randomized controlled trial testing the effect on persecutory delusions of using CBT to reduce negative cognitions about the self'. *Schizophrenia Research*, 160, 186–192.

Freeman, D., Startup, H., Dunn, G., Wingham, G., C˘ernis, E., Evans, N., Lister, R., Pugh, K., Cordwell, J. and Kingdon, D. (2014). 'Persecutory delusions and psychological well-being'. *Social Psychiatry and Psychiatric Epidemiology*, 49, 1045–1050.

Gilbert, P. (2009). 'Introducing compassion-focused therapy'. *Advances in Psychiatric Treatment*, 15(3), 199–208.

Judge, T. A. and Cable, D. M. (2004). 'The effect of physical height on workplace success and income: Preliminary test of a theoretical model'. *Journal of Applied Psychology*, 89(3), 428–441.

Lincoln, T., Hohenhaus, F. and Hartmann, M. (2013). 'Can paranoid thoughts be reduced by targeting negative emotions and self-esteem? An experimental investigation of a brief compassion-focussed intervention'. *Cognitive Therapy and Research*, 37, 390–402.

Lindqvist, E. (2012). 'Height and leadership'. *Review of Economics and Statistics*, 94(4), 1191–1196.

Marshall, E., Freeman, D. and Waite, F. (2020). 'The experience of body image concerns in patients with persecutory delusions: "People don't want to sit next to me"'. *Psychology and Psychotherapy*, 99, 639–655.

Ponzo, M. and Scoppa, V. (2015). 'Trading height for education in the marriage market'. *American Journal of Human Biology*, 27(2), 164–174.

Puhl, R. M. and Heuer, C. A. (2009). 'The stigma of obesity: A review and update'. *Obesity*, 17(5), 941–964.

Seligman, M. E. (2019). 'Positive psychology: A personal history'. *Annual Review of Clinical Psychology*, 15, 1–23.

Sheffield, J. M., Brinen, A. P. and Freeman, D. (2021). 'Paranoia and grandiosity in the general population: Differential associations with putative causal factors'. *Frontiers in Psychiatry*, 12, 668152.

Tiernan, B., Tracey, R. and Shannon, C. (2014). 'Paranoia and self-concepts in psychosis: A systematic review of the literature'. *Psychiatry Research*, 216(3), 303–313.

Vorontsova, N., Garety, P. and Freeman, D. (2013). 'Cognitive factors maintaining persecutory delusions in psychosis: The contribution of depression'. *Journal of Abnormal Psychology*, 122, 1121–1131.

Waite, F. and Freeman, D. (2017). 'Body image and paranoia'. *Psychiatry Research*, 258, 136–140.

Waite, F., Diamond, R., Collett, N., Bold, E., Chadwick, E. and Freeman, D. (2023). 'Body image concerns in patients with persecutory delusions'. *Psychological Medicine*, 53(9), 4121–4129.

Yancey, G. and Emerson, M. O. (2016). 'Does height matter? An examination of height preferences in romantic coupling'. *Journal of Family Issues*, 37(1), 53–73.

Chapter 9

Barkhuizen, W., Taylor, M. J., Freeman, D. and Ronald, A. (2019). 'A twin study on the association between psychotic experiences and tobacco use during adolescence'. *Journal of the American Academy of Child and Adolescent Psychiatry*, 58(2), 267–276.

Bell, D. A. (2015). *Napoleon:* A Concise Biography. Oxford and New York: Oxford University Press.

Carlyle, M., Constable, T., Walter, Z. C., Wilson, J., Newland, G. and Hides, L. (2021). 'Cannabis-induced dysphoria/paranoia mediates the link between childhood trauma and psychotic-like experiences in young cannabis users'. *Schizophrenia Research*, 238, 178–184.

Charles, V. and Weaver, T. (2010). 'A qualitative study of illicit and non-prescribed drug use amongst people with psychotic disorders'. *Journal of Mental Health*, 19(1), 99–106.

Childs, H. E., McCarthy-Jones, S., Rowse, G. and Turpin, G. (2011). 'The journey through cannabis use: A qualitative study of the experiences of young adults with psychosis'. *Journal of Nervous and Mental Disease*, 199(9), 703–708.

D'Souza, D. C., DiForti, M., Ganesh, S., George, T. P., Hall, W., Hjorthøj, C., Howes, O., Keshavan, M., Murray, R. M., Nguyen, T. B. and Pearlson, G. D. (2022). 'Consensus paper of the WFSBP task force on cannabis, cannabinoids and psychosis'. *World Journal of Biological Psychiatry*, 1–24.

Dai, H. and Leventhal, A. M. (2019). 'Prevalence of e-cigarette use among adults in the United States, 2014–2018'. *JAMA: The Journal of the American Medical Association*, 322(18), 1824–1827.

Doyle, P. (2019). 'Willie Nelson: The high life'. *Rolling Stone India*, rollingstoneindia.com/willie-nelson-high-life

Freeman, D., Dunn, G., Murray, R., Evans, N., Lister, R., Antley, A., Slater, M., Godlewska, B., Cornish, R., Williams, J., Di Simplicio, M., Igoumenou, A., Brenneisen, R., Tunbridge, E., Harrison, P., Harmer, C., Cowen, P. and Morrison, P. (2015). 'How cannabis causes paranoia: Using the intravenous administration of Δ9-tetrahydrocannabinol (THC) to identify key cognitive mechanisms leading to paranoia'. *Schizophrenia Bulletin*, 41, 391–399.

Freeman, D., McManus, S., Brugha, T., Meltzer, H., Jenkins, R. and Bebbington, P. (2011). 'Concomitants of paranoia in the general population'. *Psychological Medicine*, 41, 923–936.

Freeman, D., Morrison, P., Murray, R., Evans, N., Lister, R. and Dunn, G. (2013). 'Persecutory ideation and a history of cannabis use'. *Schizophrenia Research*, 148, 122–125.

Gautier, T. (1846). 'Club des haschischins'. *Revue des Deux Mondes*, urbigenous.net/library/haschischins.html

Graham, H. L., Maslin, J., Copello, A., Birchwood, M., Mueser, K., McGovern, D. and Georgiou, G. (2001). 'Drug and alcohol problems amongst individuals with severe mental health problems in an inner city area of the UK'. *Social Psychiatry and Psychiatric Epidemiology*, 36(9), 448–455.

Hickman, M., Vickerman, P., Macleod, J., Kirkbride, J. and Jones, P. B. (2007). 'Cannabis and schizophrenia: Model projections of the impact of the rise in cannabis use on historical and future trends in schizophrenia in England and Wales'. *Addiction*, 102(4), 597–606.

Israel, M. (1993). 'The rhetoric of drugs: an interview'. *Differences: A Journal of Feminist Cultural Studies*, 5(1), 1–26.

Isuru, A. and Rajasuriya, M. (2019). 'Tobacco smoking and schizophrenia: Re-examining the evidence'. *BJPsych Advances*, 25(6), 363–372.

Iversen, L. (2018). *The Science of Marijuana*. New York: Oxford University Press.

Johnstad, P. G. (2021). 'Day trip to hell: A mixed methods study of challenging psychedelic experiences'. *Journal of Psychedelic Studies*, 5(2), 114–127.

Kuipers, J., Moffa, G., Kuipers, E., Freeman, D. and Bebbington, P. (2019). 'Links between psychotic and neurotic symptoms in the general population: An analysis of longitudinal British National Survey data using Directed Acyclic Graphs'. *Psychological Medicine*, 49(3), 388–395.

Mackie, C. J., Wilson, J., Freeman, T. P., Craft, S., De La Torre, T. E. and Lynskey, M. T. (2021). 'A latent class analysis of cannabis use products in a general population sample of adolescents and their association with paranoia, hallucinations, cognitive disorganisation and grandiosity'. *Addictive Behaviors*, 117, 106837.

McManus, S., Meltzer, H. and Campion, J. (2010). 'Cigarette smoking and mental health in England: Data from the Adult Psychiatric Morbidity Survey 2007', National Centre for Social Research, natcen.ac.uk/publications/cigarette-smoking-and-mental-health-england

Office for National Statistics (2022). 'Drug misuse in England and Wales: Year ending June 2022', www.ons.gov.uk/peoplepopulatio-nandcommunity/crimeandjustice/articles/drugmisuseinenglandandwales/yearendingjune2022

Potter, D. J., Hammond, K., Tuffnell, S., Walker, C. and Di Forti, M. (2018). 'Potency of Δ9–tetrahydrocannabinol and other cannabinoids in cannabis in England in 2016: Implications for public health and pharmacology'. *Drug Testing and Analysis*, 10(4), 628–635.

Prochaska, J. J., Hall, S. M. and Bero, L. A. (2008). 'Tobacco use among individuals with schizophrenia: What role has the tobacco industry played?' *Schizophrenia Bulletin*, 34(3), 555–567.

Shakoor, S., Zavos, H. M., McGuire, P., Cardno, A. G., Freeman, D. and Ronald, A. (2015). 'Psychotic experiences are linked to cannabis use in adolescents in the community because of common underlying environmental risk factors'. *Psychiatry Research*, 227(2–3), 144–151.

Sinclair, C. (2020). *A Time to Quit: Experience of Smoking Cessation Support Among People with Severe Mental Illness.* London: Centre for Mental Health, www.rethink.org/media/3755/hwa-smi-smoking-cessation-report-2020.pdf

Substance Abuse and Mental Health Services Administration (2022). 'Key substance use and mental health indicators in the United States: Results from the 2021 National Survey on Drug Use and Health'. HHS Publication No. PEP22-07-01-005, NSDUH Series H-57. Center for Behavioral Health Statistics and Quality, Substance Abuse and Mental Health Services Administration, www.samhsa.gov/data/report/2021-nsduh-annual-national-report

Van Os, J., Bak, M., Hanssen, M., Bijl, R. V., De Graaf, R. and Verdoux, H. (2002). 'Cannabis use and psychosis: A longitudinal population-based study'. *American Journal of Epidemiology*, 156(4), 319–327.

World Health Organization (2020). 'New WHO report reveals that while smoking continues to decline among European adolescents the use of electronic cigarettes by young people is on the rise', https://www.who.int/europe/news/item/02'12-2020-new-who-report-reveals-that-while-smoking-continues-to-decline-among-european-adolescents-the-use-of-electronic-cigarettes-by-young-people-is-on the-rise

World Health Organization, Alcohol, Drugs and Addictive Behaviours Unit. 'Cannabis', www.who.int/teams/mental-health-and-substance-use/alcohol-drugs-and-addictive-behaviours/drugs-psychoactive/cannabis

Zammit, S., Allebeck, P., Andreasson, S., Lundberg, I. and Lewis, G. (2002). 'Self reported cannabis use as a risk factor for schizophrenia in Swedish conscripts of 1969: Historical cohort study'. *BMJ*, 325(7374), 1199.

Chapter 10

Bentall, R. P. (1990). 'The illusion of reality: A review and integration of psychological research on hallucinations'. *Psychological Bulletin*, 107(1), 82–95.

Chadwick, P. and Birchwood, M. (1994). 'The omnipotence of voices: A cognitive approach to auditory hallucinations'. *British Journal of Psychiatry*, 164(2), 190–201.

Grimby, A. (1993). 'Bereavement among elderly people: Grief reactions, post-bereavement hallucinations and quality of life'. *Acta Psychiatrica Scandinavica*, 87(1), 72–80.

Hurdiel, R., Monaca, C., Mauvieux, B., McCauley, P., Van Dongen, H. P. and Theunynck, D. (2012). 'Field study of sleep and functional impairments in solo sailing races'. *Sleep and Biological Rhythms*, 10(4), 270–277.

Jardri, R., Pouchet, A., Pins, D. and Thomas, P. (2011). 'Cortical activations during auditory verbal hallucinations in schizophrenia: A coordinate-based meta-analysis'. *American Journal of Psychiatry*, 168(1), 73–81.

Johns, L. C., Cannon, M., Singleton, N., Murray, R. M., Farrell, M., Brugha, T., Bebbington, P., Jenkins, R. and Meltzer, H. (2004). 'Prevalence and correlates of self-reported psychotic symptoms in the British population'. *British Journal of Psychiatry*, 185(4), 298–305.

Lennox, B. R., Park, S. B. G., Medley, I., Morris, P. G. and Jones, P. B. (2000). 'The functional anatomy of auditory hallucinations in schizophrenia'. *Psychiatry Research: Neuroimaging*, 100(1), 13–20.

Longden, E., Corstens, D., Morrison, A. P., Larkin, A., Murphy, E., Holden, N., Steele, A., Branitsky, A. and Bowe, S. (2021). 'A treatment protocol to guide the delivery of dialogical engagement with auditory hallucinations: Experience from the talking with voices pilot trial'. *Psychology and Psychotherapy*, 94(3), 558–572.

Luhrmann, T. M., Padmavati, R., Tharoor, H. and Osei, A. (2015). 'Differences in voice-hearing experiences of people with psychosis in the USA, India and Ghana: Interview-based study'. *British Journal of Psychiatry*, 206(1), 41–44.

McBain, S. (2021). 'The voice in your head'. *New Statesman*, www.newstatesman.com/politics/2021/03/voice-your-head

McGuire, P. K., Murray, R. M. and Shah, G. M. S. (1993). 'Increased blood flow in Broca's area during auditory hallucinations in schizophrenia'. *The Lancet*, 342(8873), 703–706.

Ohayon, M. M., Priest, R. G., Caulet, M. and Guilleminault, C. (1996). 'Hypnagogic and hypnopompic hallucinations: Pathological phenomena?' *British Journal of Psychiatry*, 169(4), 459–467.

Peters, E. R., Williams, S. L., Cooke, M. A. and Kuipers, E. (2012). 'It's not what you hear, it's the way you think about it: Appraisals as determinants of affect and behaviour in voice hearers'. *Psychological Medicine*, 42(7), 1507–1514.

Romme, M. A. and Escher, A. D. (1989). 'Hearing voices'. *Schizophrenia Bulletin*, 15(2), 209–216.

Rowling, J. K. (1998). *Harry Potter and the Chamber of Secrets*. London: Bloomsbury.

Sheaves, B., Johns, L., Černis, E., Griffith, L., McPin Hearing Voices Lived Experience Advisory Panel and Freeman, D. (2021). 'The challenges and opportunities of social connection when hearing derogatory and threatening voices: A thematic analysis with patients experiencing psychosis'. *Psychology and Psychotherapy*, 94, 341–356.

Sheaves, B., Johns, L., Griffith, L., Isham, L., Kabir, T. and Freeman, D. (2020). 'Why do patients with psychosis listen to and believe derogatory and threatening voices? 21 reasons given by patients'. *Behavioural and Cognitive Psychotherapy*, 48, 631–645.

Sheaves, B., Johns, L., Loe, B., Bold, E., Černis, E., The McPin Hearing Voices Lived Experience Advisory Panel, Molodynski, A. and Freeman, D. (2023). 'Listening to and believing derogatory and threatening voices'. *Schizophrenia Bulletin*, 49, 151–160.

Tsang, A., Bucci, S., Branitsky, A., Kaptan, S., Rafiq, S., Wong, S., Berry, K. and Varese, F. (2021). 'The relationship between appraisals of voices (auditory verbal hallucinations) and distress in voice-hearers with schizophrenia-spectrum diagnoses: A meta-analytic review'. *Schizophrenia Research*, 230, 38–47.

Wade, D. M., Brewin, C. R., Howell, D. C., White, E., Mythen, M. G. and Weinman, J. A. (2015). 'Intrusive memories of hallucinations and delusions in traumatized intensive care patients: an interview study'. *British Journal of Health Psychology*, 20(3), 613–631.

Waite, F., Diamond, R., Collett, N., Chadwick, E., Bold, E., Teale, A. L., Taylor, K. M., Kirkham, M., Twivy, E., Causier, C., Carr, L., Bird, J. C., Černis, E., Isham, L. and Freeman, D. (2019). 'The comments of voices on the appearance of patients with psychosis: "the voices tell me that I am ugly"'. *BJPsych Open*, 5, e86. doi: 10.1192/Čbjo.2019.66.

Chapter 11

Bacon, F., Jardine, L. and Silverthorne, M. (2000). *The New Organon*. Cambridge Texts in the History of Philosophy. Cambridge: Cambridge University Press.

Broome, M. R., Johns, L. C., Valli, I., Woolley, J. B., Tabraham, P., Brett, C., Valmaggia, L., Peters, E., Garety, P. A. and McGuire, P. K. (2007). 'Delusion formation and reasoning biases in those at clinical high risk for psychosis'. *British Journal of Psychiatry*, 191 (S51), s38–s42.

Chapman, R. K. (2002). 'First person account: Eliminating delusions'. *Schizophrenia Bulletin*, 28(3), 545–553.

Dudley, R. E. J., John, C. H., Young, A. W. and Over, D. E. (1997). 'Normal and abnormal reasoning in people with delusions'. *British Journal of Clinical Psychology*, 36(2), 243–258.

Dudley, R., Taylor, P., Wickham, S. and Hutton, P. (2016). 'Psychosis, delusions and the "jumping to conclusions" reasoning bias: A systematic review and meta-analysis'. *Schizophrenia Bulletin*, 42(3), 652–665.

Eco, U. (1980). *The Name of the Rose*. London: Vintage.

Falcone, M. A., Murray, R. M., O'Connor, J. A., Hockey, L. N., Gardner-Sood, P., Di Forti, M., Freeman, D. and Jolley, S. (2015). 'Jumping to conclusions and the persistence of delusional beliefs in first episode psychosis'. *Schizophrenia Research*, 165, 243–246.

Freeman, D., Dunn, G., Startup, H., Pugh, K., Cordwell, J., Mander, H., Černis, E., Wingham, G., Shirvell, K. and Kingdon, D. (2015). 'Effects of cognitive behaviour therapy for worry on persecutory delusions in patients with psychosis (WIT): A parallel, single-blind, randomised controlled trial with a mediation analysis'. *The Lancet Psychiatry*, 2, 305–313.

Freeman, D., Evans, N. and Lister, R. (2012). 'Gut feelings, deliberative thought, and paranoid ideation: A study of experiential and rational reasoning'. *Psychiatry Research*, 197(1–2), 119–122.

Freeman, D. and Garety, P. A. (1999). 'Worry, worry processes and dimensions of delusions: An exploratory investigation of a role for anxiety processes in the maintenance of delusional distress'. *Behavioural and Cognitive Psychotherapy*, 27, 47–62.

Freeman, D., Garety, P. A., Fowler, D., Kuipers, E., Bebbington, P. and Dunn, G. (2004). 'Why do people with delusions fail to choose more realistic explanations for their experiences? An empirical investigation'. *Journal of Consulting and Clinical Psychology*, 72, 671–680.

Freeman, D., Lister, R. and Evans, N. (2014). 'The use of intuitive and analytic reasoning styles by patients with persecutory delusions'. *Journal of Behavior Therapy and Experimental Psychiatry*, 45, 454–458.

Freeman, D., McManus, S., Brugha, T., Meltzer, H., Jenkins, R. and Bebbington, P. (2011). 'Concomitants of paranoia in the general population'. *Psychological Medicine*, 41, 923–936.

Freeman, D., Pugh, K., Antley, A., Slater, M., Bebbington, P., Gittins, M., Dunn, G., Kuipers, E., Fowler, D. and Garety, P. A. (2008). 'A virtual reality study of paranoid thinking in the general population'. *British Journal of Psychiatry*, 192, 258–263.

Freeman, D., Pugh, K. and Garety, P. (2008). 'Jumping to conclusions and paranoid ideation in the general population'. *Schizophrenia Research*, 102, 254–260.

Freeman, D., Stahl, D., McManus, S., Meltzer, H., Brugha, T., Wiles, N. and Bebbington, P. (2012). 'Insomnia, worry, anxiety and depression as predictors of the occurrence and persistence of paranoid thinking'. *Social Psychiatry and Psychiatric Epidemiology*, 47, 1195–1203.

Freeman, D., Taylor, K., Molodynski, A. and Waite, F. (2019). 'Treatable clinical intervention targets for patients with schizophrenia'. *Schizophrenia Research*, 211, 44–50.

Garety, P. A., Freeman, D., Jolley, S., Dunn, G., Bebbington, P. E., Fowler, D., Kuipers, E. and Dudley, R. (2005). 'Reasoning, emotions and delusional conviction in psychosis'. *Journal of Abnormal Psychology*, 114, 373–384.

Garety, P. A. and Hemsley, D. R. (1994). *Delusions: Investigations Into the Psychology of Delusional Reasoning*. Oxford: Oxford University Press.

Garety, P. A., Hemsley, D. and Wessely, S. (1991) 'Reasoning in deluded schizophrenic and paranoid subjects: Biases in performance on a probabilistic inference task'. *Journal of Nervous and Mental Disease*, 179, 194–201.

Garety, P., Waller, H., Emsley, R., Jolley, S., Kuipers, E., Bebbington, P., Dunn, G., Fowler, D., Hardy, A. and Freeman, D. (2015). 'Cognitive mechanisms of change in delusions'. *Schizophrenia Bulletin*, 41, 400–410.

Garety, P., Ward, T., Emsley, R., Greenwood, K., Freeman, D., Fowler, D., Kuipers, E., Bebbington, P., Rus-Calafell, M., McGourty, A., Sacadura, C., Collett, N., James, K. and Hardy, A. (2021). 'Effects of SlowMo, a blended digital therapy targeting reasoning, on paranoia among people with psychosis: a randomized clinical trial'. *JAMA Psychiatry*, 78, 714–725.

Greenwood, K. E., Gurnani, M., Ward, T., Vogel, E., Vella, C., McGourty, A., Robertson, S., Sacadura, C., Hardy, A., Rus-Calafell,

M., Collett, N., Emsley, R., Freeman, D., Fowler, D., Kuipers, E., Bebbington, P., Dunn, G., Michelson, D., Garety, P. and SlowMo Patient, Public Involvement (PPI) team (2022). 'The service user experience of SlowMo therapy: A co-produced thematic analysis of service users' subjective experience'. *Psychology and Psychotherapy*, 95(3), 680–700.

Hardy, A., Wojdecka, A., West, J., Matthews, E., Golby, C., Ward, T., Lopez, N. D., Freeman, D., Waller, H., Kuipers, E., Bebbington, P., Fowler, D., Emsley, R., Dunn, G. and Garety, P. (2018). 'How inclusive, user-centered design research can improve psychological therapies for psychosis: Development of SlowMo. *JMIR Mental Health*, 5:e11222.

Henquet, C., Van Os, J., Pries, L. K., Rauschenberg, C., Delespaul, P., Kenis, G., Luykx, J. J., Lin, B. D., Richards, A. L., Akdede, B. and Binbay, T. (2022). 'A replication study of JTC bias, genetic liability for psychosis and delusional ideation'. *Psychological Medicine*, 52, 1777–1783.

Kahneman, D. (2011). *Thinking, Fast and Slow*. London: Macmillan.

Nickerson, R. S. (1998). 'Confirmation bias: A ubiquitous phenomenon in many guises'. *Review of General Psychology*, 2(2), 175–220.

Peters, E. and Garety, P. (2006). 'Cognitive functioning in delusions: A longitudinal analysis'. *Behaviour Research and Therapy*, 44(4), 481–514.

Ross, K., Freeman, D., Dunn, G. and Garety, P. (2011). 'Can jumping to conclusions be reduced in people with delusions? An experimental investigation of a brief reasoning training module'. *Schizophrenia Bulletin*, 37, 324–333.

Startup, H., Pugh, K., Dunn, G., Cordwell, J., Mander, H., Černis, E., Wingham, G., Shirvell, K., Kingdon, D. and Freeman, D. (2016). 'Worry processes in patients with persecutory delusions'. *British Journal of Clinical Psychology*, 55, 387–400.

Waller, H., Freeman, D., Jolley, S., Dunn, G. and Garety, P. (2011). 'Targeting reasoning biases in delusions'. *Journal of Behavior Therapy and Experimental Psychiatry*, 42, 414–421.

Ward, T. and Garety, P. A. (2019). 'Fast and slow thinking in distressing delusions: A review of the literature and implications for targeted therapy'. *Schizophrenia Research*, 203, 80–87.

Wason, P. C. (1960). 'On the failure to eliminate hypotheses in a conceptual task'. *Quarterly Journal of Experimental Psychology*, 12, 129–140.

Chapter 12

Altunkaya, J., Craven, M., Lambe, S., Beckley, A., Rosebrock, L., Dudley, R., Chapman, K., Morrison, A., O'Regan, E., Grabey, J., Bergin, A., Kabir, T., Waite, F., Freeman, D. and Leal, J. (2022). 'Estimating the economic value of automated virtual reality cognitive therapy for treating agoraphobic avoidance in patients with psychosis: Findings from the gameChange randomized controlled clinical trial'. *Journal of Medical Internet Research*, 24(11) e39248.

Bond, J., Kenny, A., Pinfold, V., Couperthwaite, L., gamChange Lived Experience Advisory Panel, Kabir, T., Larkin, M., Petit, A., Rosebrock, L., Lambe, S., Freeman, D., Waite, F. and Robotham, D. (2023). 'A safe place to learn: A peer research qualitative investigation of automated virtual reality cognitive therapy (gameChange)'. *JMIR Serious Games*. Jan 16, e38065.

Brown, P., Waite, F., Lambe, S., Rosebrock, L. and Freeman, D. (2020). 'Virtual reality cognitive therapy in inpatient psychiatric wards: Protocol for a qualitative investigation of staff and patient views across multiple National Health Service sites'. *JMIR Research Protocols*, 9(8), e20300.

Bruner, J. (1983). 'Play, thought, and language'. *Peabody Journal of Education*, 60(3), 60–69.

Freeman, D., Lambe, S., Galal, U., Yu, L.-M., Kabir, T., Petit, A., Rosebrock, L., Dudley, R., Chapman, K., Morrison, A., O'Regan, E., Murphy, E., Aynsworth, C., Jones, J., Powling, R., Grabey, J., Rovira, A., Freeman, J., Clark, D. M. and Waite, F. (2022). 'Agoraphobic avoidance in patients with psychosis: Severity and response to automated VR therapy in a secondary analysis of a randomised controlled clinical trial'. *Schizophrenia Research*, 250, 50–59.

Freeman, D., Lambe, S., Kabir, T., Petit, A., Rosebrock, L., Yu, L.-M., Dudley, R., Chapman, K., Morrison, A., O'Regan, E., Aynsworth, C., Jones, J., Murphy, E., Powling, R., Galal, U., Grabey, J., Rovira, A., Martin, J., Hollis, C., Clark, D. M., Waite, F. and gameChange Trial Group (2022). 'Automated virtual reality therapy to treat agoraphobic avoidance and distress in patients with psychosis (gameChange): A multicentre, parallel-group, single-blind, randomised, controlled trial in England with mediation and moderation analyses'. *The Lancet Psychiatry*, 9, 375–388.

Freeman, D., Rosebrock, L., Waite, F., Loe, B. S., Kabir, T., Petit, A., Dudley, R., Chapman, K., Morrison, A., O'Regan, E., Aynsworth, C., Jones, J., Murphy, E., Powling, R., Peel, H., Walker, H., Byrne, R., Freeman, J., Rovira, A., Galal, U., Yu, L.-M., Clark, D. M. and Lambe, S. (2023). 'Virtual reality (VR) therapy for patients with psychosis: satisfaction and side effects'. *Psychological Medicine*, 53, 4373–4384.

Freeman, D., Taylor, K., Molodynski, A. and Waite, F. (2019). 'Treatable clinical intervention targets for patients with schizophrenia'. *Schizophrenia Research*, 211, 44–50.

Gelder, M. G. and Marks, I. M. (1966). 'Severe agoraphobia: A controlled prospective trial of behaviour therapy'. *British Journal of Psychiatry*, 112, 309–319.

Knight, I., West, J., Matthews, E., Kabir, T., Lambe, S., Waite, F. and Freeman, D. (2021). 'Participatory design to create a VR therapy for psychosis'. *Design for Health*, 5, 98–119.

Lambe, S., Bird, J., Loe, B., Rosebrock, L., Kabir, T., Petit, A., Mulhall, S., Jenner, L., Aynsworth, C., Murphy, E., Jones, J., Powling, R., Chapman, K., Dudley, R., Morrison, A., O'Regan, E., Yu, L.-M., Clark, D., Waite, F. and Freeman, D. (2023). 'The Oxford Agoraphobic Avoidance Scale'. *Psychological Medicine*, 53, 1233–1243.

Lambe, S., Knight, I., Kabir, T., West, J., Patel, R., Lister, R., Rosebrock, L., Rovira, A., Garnish, B., Freeman, J., Clark, D. M.,

Waite, F. and Freeman, D. (2020). 'Developing an automated VR cognitive treatment for psychosis: gameChange VR therapy'. *Journal of Behavioural and Cognitive Therapy*, 30, 33–40.

Lanier, J. (2017). *Dawn of the New Everything: A Journey Through Virtual Reality*. London: Bodley Head.

Rosebrock, L., Lambe, S., Mulhall, S., Petit, A., Loe, B. S., Saidel, S., Pervez, M., Mitchell, J., Chauhan, N., Prouten, E., Chan, C., Aynsworth, C., Murphy, E., Jones, J., Powling, R., Chapman, K., Dudley, R., Morrison, A., O'Regan, E., Clark, D. M., Waite, F. and Freeman, D. (2022). 'Understanding agoraphobic avoidance: The development of the Oxford Cognitions and Defences Questionnaire (O-DCQ)'. *Behavioural and Cognitive Psychotherapy*, 50, 257–268.

Wei, S., Freeman, D. and Rovira, A. (2023). 'A randomised controlled test of emotional attributes of a virtual coach within a virtual reality (VR) mental health treatment'. *Scientific Reports*, 13(1), 11517.

Chapter 13

Alshuibani, A., Shevlin, M., Freeman, D., Sheaves, B. and Bentall, R. (2022). 'Why conspiracy theorists are not always paranoid: Conspiracy theories and paranoia form separate factors with distinct psychological predictors'. *PLoS One*, 17: e0259053.

BBC News (2020). 'Coronavirus: WHO chief warns against "trolls and conspiracy theories"', www.bbc.co.uk/news/world-51429400

Brotherton, R., French, C. and Pickering, A. (2013). 'Measuring Belief in Conspiracy Theories: The Generic Conspiracist Beliefs Scale'. *Frontiers in Psychology*, 4, 279.

Brown, P., Waite, F., Larkin, M., Lambe, S., McShane, H., Pollard, A. J. and Freeman, D. (2022). '"It seems impossible that it's been made so quickly": A qualitative investigation of concerns about the speed of COVID-19 vaccine development and how these may be overcome'. *Human Vaccines and Immunotherapeutics*, 18:1, 2004808.

Burki, T. (2021). 'Increasing COVID-19 vaccine uptake in Black

Americans'. *The Lancet Infectious Diseases*, 21(11), 1500–1501.

Chadwick, A., Kaiser, J., Vaccari, C., Freeman, D., Lambe, S., Loe, B. S., Vanderslott, S., Lewandowsky, S., Conroy, M., Ross, A., Innocenti, S., Pollard, A., Waite, F., Larkin, M., Rosebrock, L., Jenner, L., McShane, H., Giubilini, A., Petit, A. and Yu, L.-M. (2021). 'Online social endorsement and Covid-19 vaccine hesitancy in the UK'. *Social Media and Society*, 7 (2), 20563051211008817.

Chadwick, A. and Vaccari, C. (2019). 'News sharing on UK social media: misinformation, disinformation, and correction'. Loughborough University.

Devlin, H. (2023). 'London at risk of major measles outbreak, UK Health Security Agency warns'. *Guardian*, www.theguardian.com/society/2023/jul/14/measles-outbreak-risk-london-uk-health-secu-rity-agency-mmr-vaccine-take-up

Fazel, M., Puntis, S., White, S., Townsend, A., Mansfield, K., Viner, R., Herring, J., Pollard, A. and Freeman, D. (2021). 'Willingness of children and adolescents to have a COVID-19 vaccination: Results of a large whole schools survey in England'. *EClinicalMedicine*, Sep 27, 101144.

Freeman, D. and Bentall, R. (2017). 'The concomitants of conspiracy concerns'. *Social Psychiatry and Psychiatric Epidemiology*, 52, 595–604.

Freeman, D., Loe, B. S., Chadwick, A., Vaccari, C., Waite, F., Rosebrock, L., Jenner, L., Petit, A., Lewandowsky, S., Vanderslott, S., Innocenti, S., Larkin, M., Giubilini, A., Yu, L.-M., McShane, H., Pollard, A. J. and Lambe, S. (2022). 'COVID-19 vaccine hesitancy in the UK: The Oxford Coronavirus Explanations, Attitudes, and Narratives Survey (OCEANS II) *Psychological Medicine*, 52, 3127-3141.

Freeman, D., Loe, B. S., Yu, L.M., Freeman, J., Chadwick, A., Vaccari, C., Shanyinde, M., Harris, V., Waite, F., Rosebrock, L., Petit, A., Vanderslott, S., Lewandowsky, S., Larkin, M., Innocenti, S., Pollard, A., McShane, H. and Lambe, S. (2021). 'Effects of different types of written vaccination information on COVID-19 vaccine hesitancy in the UK (OCEANS-III): A single-blind, parallel-group, randomised controlled trial'. *The Lancet Public Health*, 6, E416–427.

Freeman, D., Waite, F., Rosebrock, L., Petit, A., Causier, C., East, A., Jenner, L., Teale, A., Carr, L., Mulhall, S., Bold, E. and Lambe, S. (2022). 'Coronavirus conspiracy beliefs, mistrust, and compliance with government guidelines in England'. *Psychological Medicine*, 52, 251–263.

Goertzel, T. (1994). 'Belief in conspiracy theories'. *Political Psychology*, 15, 731–742.

Imhoff, R. and Bruder, M. (2014). 'Speaking (un-)truth to power: Conspiracy mentality as a generalized political attitude'. *European Journal of Personality*, 28, 25–43.

Lewandowsky, S., Oberauer, K. and Gignac, G. E. (2013). 'NASA faked the moon landing – therefore, (climate) science is a hoax: An anatomy of the motivated rejection of science'. *Psychological Science*, 24(5), 622–633.

Martinez, A. P., Shevlin, M., Valiente, C., Hyland, P. and Bentall, R. P. (2022). 'Paranoid beliefs and conspiracy mentality are associated with different forms of mistrust: A three-nation study'. *Frontiers in Psychology*, 13, 1023366.

Neuman, N. (2022). 'Overview and key findings of the 2022 Digital News Report'. Reuters Institute, reutersinstitute.politics.ox.ac.uk/digital-news-report/2022/dnr-executive-summary

New York Times (2020; 2022). 'See how vaccinations are going in your county and state', www.nytimes.com/interactive/2020/us/covid-19-vaccine-doses.html

Office for National Statistics (2023). 'Coronavirus (COVID-19) latest insights: Vaccines'. Office for National Statistics, www.ons.gov.uk/peoplepopulationandcommunity/healthandsocialcare/conditionsanddiseases/articles/coronaviruscovid19latestinsights/vaccines

Oxford Vaccine Group (2022). 'Measles'. University of Oxford, vk.ovg.ox.ac.uk/vk/measles

Petrosyan, A. (2023). 'Average daily time spent using media in the United Kingdom (UK) in the 3rd quarter 2022'. Statista, www.statista.com/statistics/507378/average-daily-media-use-in-the-united-kingdom-uk/

Shacle, S. (2021). 'Among the Covid sceptics: "We are being manipulated, without a shadow of a doubt"'. *Guardian*, www.theguardian.com/news/2021/apr/08/among-covid-sceptics-we-are-being-manipulated-anti-lockdown

Sunstein, C. R. and Vermeule, C. A. (2009). 'Conspiracy theories: Causes and cures'. *Journal of Political Philosophy*, 17, 202–227.

Swami, V., Chamorro-Premuzic, T. and Furnham, A. (2010). 'Unanswered questions: A preliminary investigation of personality and individual difference predictors of 9/11 conspiracist beliefs'. *Applied Cognitive Psychology*, 24, 749–761.

Torracinta, L., Tanner, R. and Vanderslott, S. (2021). 'MMR vaccine attitude and uptake research in the United Kingdom: A critical review'. *Vaccines*, 9(4), 402.

Uscinski, J. E. (2018). *Conspiracy Theories and the People Who Believe Them*. New York: Oxford University Press.

Wood, M. J., Douglas, K. M. and Sutton, R. M. (2012). 'Dead and alive'. *Social Psychological and Personality Science*, 3(6), 767–773.

World Health Organization (2020). 'Immunizing the public against misinformation', www.who.int/news-room/feature-stories/detail/immunizing-the-public-against-misinformation

Chapter 14

Freeman, D. (2023). 'The Phoenix virtual reality self-confidence study'. ISRCTN registry, www.isrctn.com/ISRCTN10250113

Freeman, D., Freeman, J., Ahmed, M., Haynes, P., Beckwith, H., Rovira, A., Miguel, A. L., Ward, R., Bousfield, M., Riffiod, L., Kabir, T., Waite, F. and Rosebrock, L. (in press). 'Automated VR therapy for improving positive self beliefs and psychological wellbeing in young patients with psychosis: A proof of concept evaluation of Phoenix VR self-confidence therapy'. *Behavioural and Cognitive Psychotherapy*.

Harding, L. (2022). *Invasion: Russia's Bloody War and Ukraine's Fight for Survival*. London: Guardian Faber.

Hoffman, D. (2009). *The Dead Hand: Reagan, Gorbachev and the Story of the Cold War Arms Race*. London: Icon Books.

Meek, J. (2020). 'Red pill, blue pill'. *London Review of Books*, www.lrb.co.uk/the-paper/v42/n20/james-meek/red-pill-blue-pill

MQ (n.d.). 'UK mental health research funding 2014–2017', MQ Mental Health Research, www.mqmentalhealth.org/wp-content/uploads/UKMentalHealthResearchFunding2014-2017digital.pdf

Reagan, R. (1983). 'Evil Empire speech'. Voices of Democracy, voicesofdemocracy.umd.edu/reagan-evil-empire-speech-text/

Taylor, M. (2022). 'We cannot continue to neglect mental health funding'. NHS Confederation, www.nhsconfed.org/articles/we-can-not-continue-neglect-mental-health-funding#:~:text=Lack%20of%20funding%20is%20risking%20progress&text=Yet%20only%20about%20a%20third,per%20cent%20of%20NHS%20spending

Tolmeijer, E., Waite, F., Isham, L., Bringmann, L., Timmers, R., van den Berg, A., Schuurmans, H., Staring, A. P. B., de Bont, P., van Grunsven, R., Stulp, G., Wijnen, B., van der Gaag, M., Freeman, D. and van den Berg, D. (manuscript submitted for publication). 'Testing the combination of Feeling Safe and peer counselling against formulation-based cognitive behavior therapy to promote psychological wellbeing in people with persecutory delusions: Study protocol for a randomized controlled trial (the Feeling Safe-NL Trial)'.

US Department of State (2020). 'Communist China and the free world's future: Secretary Pompeo at the Nixon Memorial Library', www.youtube.com/watch?v=7azj-t0gtPM

Van den Berg, D. and Tolmeijer, E. (2022). 'Feeling Safe-Netherlands: Recovery-oriented cognitive behaviour therapy to promote well-being and feeling safer'. IRSCTN registry, www.isrctn.com/ISRCTN25766661

Index

Tables are indicated by the use of *italic* page numbers.